ILLUMINATING

PHILOSOPHY

STORIES

BEYOND

BOUNDARIES

SAMUEL GOROVITZ

Prospecta Press

Paperback ISBN 978-1-63226-129-8
eBook ISBN 978-1-63226-130-4

Prospecta Press
PO Box 3131
Westport CT 06880
(203) 571-0781

www.prospectapress.com

Book and cover design by Alexia Garaventa

Manufactured in the United States of America

This book is dedicated to you, the reader, in appreciation for your being a reader of books and in hope that this one prompts you to agree or disagree with what I have said, and to discuss it with others as you see fit.

CONTENTS

FOREWORD

Arthur L. Caplan

If you know Sam Gorovitz even a tiny bit, you will know that he uses language very carefully and precisely. Thus, in thinking about the title he chose for this engaging and insightful collection of essays, one wants to pay careful attention to the words he picked, especially "illuminating" and "boundaries."

So I consulted a few dictionaries, suspecting that Sam would have done so in choosing his title. "Illuminate" turns out to have three main definitions. The first is "to brighten with light," which explains the Latin origin of this verb—*illuminare*—to light up.

Readers of this book, if they follow Sam's bright intellectual torch, will rapidly appreciate the obscure, hard-to-see nooks and conceptual crannies explored in these essays. Often one might say the argument or the insight lies in the nuanced details, not, as he warns, in the rote application of a rule or algorithm.

"Illuminate" also means to clarify or explain. Sam is a master at this task, offering historical exegesis of the origins of his thinking about philosophy and bioethics on to contemporary debates about authenticity and provenance in the arts and by analogy in many other areas of life. It is authenticity and history that, he makes clear, shape many of our evaluations.

He also explains how, in the conceptual thicket that characterizes so many contemporary ethical challenges, or in seeking to bridge yawning ideological divides, we ought to seek to persuade. Sam demonstrates that this involves identifying key claims, organizing an argument, and marshalling evidence for or against the claims of the argument: pragmatic critical thinking made clear.

"Illuminate" also can be used to describe decorating a page, letter, or a book with colorful designs and illustrations, such as you can find in *The Book of Kells*, the *Grimani Breviary*, or the *Black Hours*. Look them up online, they are amazing.

But, you are probably thinking, this book has no illustrations, artwork, doodles (Sam explicitly notes he is doodle-impaired), or pictures. True, but this is where boundaries come in.

This book is a wonderful example of crossing boundaries to illuminate points, using word-pictures, analogies, metaphors, and ideas drawn (pun intended) from poetry, literature, baseball, religion, paintings, museum displays, music, and many other intellectual domains. Want to capture someone's attention with an argument? Watch a master "idea" painter lure you in with examples and illuminations of his stories from a huge swath of intellectual life.

There is a deeper point to be garnered from the stories told here. It has become popular in many circles from the *Economist* magazine to scholars such as the distinguished American economist Bryan Caplan, to wonder if college is worth the money. What those asking the question or answering "no" do is to look at the incomes of college graduates relative to the money they paid to attend. For many students, the answer is that they are paying too much. If they had jump-started a career without college they would be far ahead in terms of income and advancement relative to their degree-seeking peers.

There is some truth to this argument. College often does cost too much, with rates that leave too many students and/or their families in serious debt. Worse, many colleges are outright scams, promising learning and jobs but delivering neither. From Trump University to Corinthian Colleges to even the giant University of Phoenix, for-profit colleges are simply engines of profits for investors.

The U.S. Senate has found that the federal student loan program is "plagued by fraud and abuse." Their examination of the industry heaped special scorn on for-profit trade schools for serving 22 percent of federal student loan borrowers but accounting for 44 percent of defaults.

Scams and prices aside, what is missed in these arguments about the earning power of a college degree is the value of learning history, provenance, culture, skepticism, and critical thinking. Sure, one hopes for a lucrative job post-college or even without college, but what is one to do with one's money? Presumably spend it to obtain sustenance as well as enjoy it. But as Socrates famously warned, "The unexamined life is not worth living." If you don't acquire the skills and knowledge to think hard about your life and what you want to do with it—through a college education that is broader than vocational training or acquiring saleable skills, or perhaps through self-study, mentoring, or similarly rich experiences—then how are you to do what this book's author very much wants you to do, which is to appreciate the diversity of the world, its history, the achievements of its finest minds, and the failures of its worst, and to think hard and thoughtfully with sound judgment about how to live best in it? Is college worth it? If it can position a person to be better able to do that, then most likely it is. Is this book an invaluable tool to provision as a part of your life's self-reflective journey? Most certainly it is.

PREFACE

Creativity is often fueled by blending ideas, images, perceptions, or processes that initially seem unrelated. I'm convinced that any two items we name are related to each other if we can see deeply and imaginatively enough to recognize, or invent, the relationships. In revealing the unexpected connections in the stories told here, I'm exploring the wellsprings of creativity as well as other through-going themes. These stories draw on more than sixty years of my unusually fortunate academic life as a philosopher interacting with people within and beyond academia. Stories may be heartbreaking, distracting, funny, shocking, inspiring, revealing, and sometimes unforgettable. Here's why these twenty-five stories are worth telling:

In clinical research, rigorous experimental methods are essential. This typically requires randomized controls and robust statistical analysis. But even at its rare best, that reveals only part of what we strive to understand. No two patients are identical, so case reports—the stories of specific individuals—are crucial for medical investigation. Telling the stories of specific cases and exploring the related contexts, causes, conflicts, outcomes, and values has been fundamental to medical progress. Bioethics also relies on stories to go beyond the arid analysis of principles and codes, to deepen our understanding by considering the lived experiences of specific people in difficult situations. Two of my early books (*Doctors' Dilemmas: Moral Conflict and Medical Care* and *Drawing the Line: Life, Death and Ethical Choices in an American Hospital*) do precisely that. Considering hypothetical stories is familiar in philosophy; two classic examples are Philippa Foot's story about a trolley problem and Judy Jarvis Thomson's story about a violinist attached to a hospital patient. Those fictional stories can help clarify our values and reasoning. But the most powerful stories are about real people and their actual experiences.

During an extended visit at Boston's Beth Israel Hospital, as a writer attached to the president's office, I witnessed one case discussed separately by surgeons and by internists. No one else attended both sessions. There was scant overlap in content, and no similarity in judgment about appropriate treatment. Remarkably different claims were made about the care of that patient. Knowing that it was the same patient taught me an unforgettable lesson about the perils of an inquiry limited to like-minded people. During the Covid-19 lockdown, we heard stories from celebrities, custodians, political leaders, bus drivers, children, grandparents, and pretty much everyone else—stories that helped us understand better what it was like to be that person. There's no substitute for learning what it's like to be someone else, to see the world as that other person does, and to reevaluate our own views in light of that learning. True stories can enable us to do this. The stories here—some long, many very short, and often surprising—illuminate deep features of human character and difficult choices, of social structures, of intellectual creativity, and of the bogus boundaries that can impose a repressive mindset on the typical thinking in any one domain. This book also draws on several of my recent scholarly publications on interdisciplinary mentoring (https://www.insidehighered.com/advice/2019/05/07/importance-interdisciplinary-scholarly-mentoring-opinion) and on confronting and overcoming racism and sexism in medicine (https://surface.syr.edu/syracuse_unbound/1/)—work that caused me to revisit other case reports from my own history as a writer, academic project leader, and dean of a large college of arts and sciences.

As an undergraduate I delighted in disciplinary diversity. I especially savored seeking connections among fields often considered unrelated. It was a privilege to be exposed in classes at MIT to excellence at the highest levels—linguistics with Noam Chomsky, physics with Victor Weisskopf, engineering design with Tom Sheridan, literature with Norman Holland (a former electrical engineer and patent attorney)—all with broad interdisciplinary perspectives. Outside of class, the atmosphere also sizzled with enriching encounters: Norbert Wiener warned us not to become victims of accounting systems we devise to help us; Harold ("Doc") Edgerton made clear that his work as a scientist, engineer, and acclaimed artist were all of a piece, not the juxtaposition of multiple personae, but one integrated outlook incorporating all those dimensions in each endeavor. The treasured MIT tradition of elaborate and technically sophisticated pranks that sometimes took years to plan and dedicated teams to implement was part of that atmosphere. I started collecting stories there, and then.

These chapters interact with one another, involve brief events or prolonged developments, and feature both famous names and ordinary folks whose names are lost to memory. Throughout, they reveal unexpected connections, illuminate creativity, and probe the enigmatic question of what constitutes good judgment. The stories include my recent work on the Covid-19 pandemic (https://onlinelibrary.wiley.com/doi/10.1002/hast.1117), and go back to the unexpected opportunity, in 1957, to ask the renowned physicist Niels Bohr about modern art.

$$\left(1 \right)$$

APPROACHING
FROM ABOVE

The U-2 has provided intelligence during operations in Korea, the Balkans, Afghanistan, and Iraq. When requested, the U-2 also provides peacetime reconnaissance in support of disaster relief from floods, earthquakes, and forest fires as well as search and rescue operations.

—US Air Force Fact Sheet (2023)

Everyone who travels much by air has abundant stories—of missed connections, lost luggage, double-booking of assigned seats, overbooking, duplicitous cabin announcements, inexplicable last-minute cancellations or rerouting, extended unexplained delays, hours of imprisonment on the tarmac, and more. Inside a commercial airliner, one finds a world of its own, a separate place replete with distinctive risks and opportunities. I don't mean the illusory risk of flying that some people fear. With about sixteen million domestic flights each year, and a nearly perfect air safety record year after year, commercial airlines are less dangerous than the drive to the airport to take the flight. I mean the risks *within* the flight.

It's distressing to have one's seat kicked repeatedly from behind by a child with a distracted or indifferent parent, to have the passenger directly in front immediately push the seat back into one's scant space, or to have the adjacent vacant seat filled at the last moment by someone marinated in garlic and reeking of tobacco. I once even had an arriving seat-neighbor ask me to raise the armrest between our seats because the unfortunate fellow was too obese to fit into his own seat and he wanted to overflow into my all-too-narrow space.

Those are minor annoyances. The perils most feared are conversational. I did not want to offend or hurt the feelings of an unrelenting evangelical proselytizer who thought saving my soul was the best use of his time in flight, but perhaps I did so when I feigned a need to work in conditions that made actually getting any work done impossible. And I regretted replying honestly about my work to another earnest passenger who, hearing that one of my areas is bioethics, launched impassioned rants about every medical mishap, one by one, that had afflicted any member of her extended family—and sought advice about remedies for each one. A colleague of mine—a distinguished M.D./bioethicist—so tired of this phenomenon that she started claiming on flights to be a grocery store clerk.

It's not much safer to admit to being a philosopher. In-flight conversations often include the question, "What do you do?" If I reply that I am a philosopher, reactions range from the rare glimmer of recognition, through puzzlement, to occasional stark terror. I explain as well as I can, and some-times am rewarded by signs of comprehension. Yet the level of public understanding of what philosophers do—even among the college-educated, is subterranean. (The contrast is vivid if I talk about administrative work, like overseeing a college of arts and sciences with seven hundred people on the payroll and laboratories of many kinds. They understand that; that's real, almost like business. But I am getting ahead of the story.)

A common usage of "philosophy" is akin to "opinion"—as in, "Well, my philosophy about composting is . . ." Admitting to being a philosopher can prompt a torrent of opinion about anything on a passenger's mind, producing my heartfelt yearning for the comfort of silence (about which more later). Some seating-neighbors had encountered academic phi-losophy as an imposed requirement of their schooling, of which they consider themselves unrecovered victims. I do my best to explain that they're not cognitively deficient but were exposed to inappropriate teaching that misrepresented the field and suppressed their own capacity for creative and reflective thinking.

Lest I seem too grumpy, I acknowledge many positive encounters. I've had lively conversations with people from whom I've learned, and I've had some gratifying opportu-nities to help fellow passengers. One woman was rigid with fear, never having flown before. I said, "You'll be fine," and silently took her hand. She gripped mine tightly and held on, eyes closed, until we were at altitude. Then she turned to me, smiled, took a deep breath, released my hand, and said, "Thank you so much." That was decades ago; I can still see that smile.

Being flanked by empty seats is ideal, but rare. Those beside me are often sociable, but not always. Once, on a flight from Hamburg to London, a large, ruddy, thoroughly nineteenth-century Englishman next to me was anything but sociable. He did not speak to me and when spoken to replied with a peremptory grunt. Only when our imminent landing was announced did he become verbal. "I say," he harrumphed, "Do you happen to know, when we approach Heathrow Airport, from which direction will we approach it?" "Yes, I do know," I replied as he leaned forward eagerly. "We will approach it from above." As he withdrew in silent dismay, I thought, "That will teach you to fly so unsociably, next to a philosopher." Although I did not realize it in the moment, I'd been accustomed for decades to zoom out to a high altitude, survey the broad context, look for relationships among things that seemed disparate when viewed at close hand, and try to see with the richer perspective of what today might be called a drone's eye view.

My interest in philosophy was helped along, perhaps even began, when I read Plato in high school. The English teacher, Dr. Campbell, respected our ability to appreciate difficult primary sources, and he also enjoyed a good prank. My college experience was chaotic; starting in mechanical engineering, I lurched from one discipline to another, my interests apparently evolving as a function of what I seemed good or bad at, and of what influence my teachers had. I cannot overemphasize the influence of those teachers. Most were adequate or good, a few deeply awful, some simply annoying, and remarkably many were powerfully inspiring. Nearly all those powerful sources of inspiration were non-philosophers. They taught history, literature, classics, linguistics, mathematics, physics, and even mechanical engineering. Some were figures of great renown, others little known outside MIT.

Each, in some way—and their ways were quite different—injected distinctive excitement into my undergraduate days. Some were brilliant lecturers, others impressed with unremitting kindness and concern. One invited our class home to dinner. We loved being in that gracious home, eating good food, engaging in mature conversation, and acting uncharacteristically refined! Another, in a Western Civilization class of thirty sophomores, brought a guest one day. He announced, "We have a visitor. We won't follow the syllabus. He won't lecture but will be happy to talk with you and answer any questions you have. This is Niels Bohr." That magical hour brought an intense excitement that lingers still.

Two professors, as different as could be, taught a class together: one, an irreverent, iconoclastic cynic, the other a meticulously traditional classical scholar. "You may, of course, Ladies and Gentlemen, disagree with Aristotle in various places where you feel that you must. But always, always, with the utmost respect," cautioned the latter. Later he explained, "Plotinus puzzled about whether the forms were instantiated in, as it were, an undifferentiated substratum of existence, or whether, instead, a rather more specifically defined substratum, so to speak, were required, as in the case of, for example, say, a horse, which ah, could only be instantiated in, in, ah, as it were, in . . ." And the other professor interrupted, "In horsemeat, Harold, in horsemeat." I became enamored of collaborative teaching (with professors who are not merely juxtaposed, but genuinely interacting) and have often co-taught ever since.

The net impact of all this was to convince me that a university environment was more fun than I could imagine any other to be. I think I first wanted to be a professor of some sort, without clarity about what field to pursue. I enjoyed writing and wasn't bad at it—better at least than I was at some of the most challenging technical material. In physics, for example, it wasn't that I couldn't get the right answer. It was that even when I did get the right answer, I didn't do it as those destined to be physicists did. Which of the many mathematically correct solutions to an equation is of significance to the physics problem represented by the equation? Some people just knew, apparently intuitively, whereas I just ground out solutions.

Years later I saw a parallel phenomenon on the ski slopes of the Berner Oberland and remembered some of my especially talented physics and mathematics classmates. I knew the Swiss ski instructors would ski better than I ever could. But I noticed with surprise and perhaps some resentment that they could even just stand around better than I could! It was a matter of grace, of being completely natural and at ease in the context—of having been good at it as long as they could remember. That's how it was with the naturally gifted physicists and mathematicians. I was no more one of them than I was a potential ski instructor.

Philosophy offered the appeal of "the big questions." So did literature and drama. But I liked the rigor of philosophy, which I saw as a somewhat less radical abandonment of the technical path I had begun. Most appealing of all was that the philosopher's agenda seemed totally open and unconstrained because whatever anyone was interested in, one could inquire into the philosophy of *that*. The various styles and ways of knowing in the different disciplines provided an intriguing juxtaposition of intellectual differences, about which I wanted to learn more.

I wrote a senior thesis on the role of intuition in mathematics and ethics. I doubt it amounted to much, but the painful experience of writing it under stringent tutelage taught me a lesson that has served me superbly ever since: a good fourth draft, much improved over the third draft, is not good enough if there is any way to make a fifth draft better. There was no option to major in philosophy at MIT then, but my academic accumulations enabled me to emerge with a degree in "Humanities and Science." Armed with that, and with the advantage of having survived six semesters of physics and eight of mathematics, I went to graduate school in philosophy, interested from the outset in its application to other realms of thought and practice.

It's a challenge for any writer to know how long to struggle with a work and when to send it forth with all the prospects for praise and denigration that attend public exposure. How risk-averse a writer is depends partly on the height of the writer's standards and partly on the degree of confidence, or insecurity, or thin-skin, or objectives of that writer. I watched the full range. One of my professors withheld stunningly good pieces from public view for years on end. Another, whose assistant I was for a time, had a style more suggestive of the corporate executive than of Mr. Chips. I saw him stride into his office one day, turn to his secretary, say "Louise, take an article," and start a prolonged dictation, without notes, that yielded a complete draft. (His articles flowed forth abundantly and were good.) It was years before I was comfortable with my own approach to thinking of a work as finished. At some point I realized that I was more interested in advancing the inquiry than in being seen as getting everything exactly right. (I grant that the former is easier to do than the latter.)

There wasn't much about graduate school that I didn't like, and the rigors and diversity of my undergraduate training helped me get through it swiftly. My writing then was more the work of one wanting to join the club than one with fresh ideas about what sort of club it should be. I suppose I had some independence of mind even then, however. Graduate school has only limited tolerance for deviant interests; a few of my colleagues and faculty thought it odd that I took a course in literature when no other doctoral student took any course outside the department that was not specifically related to the doctoral program. (Yet it seemed so obvious: the great Malcolm Cowley was teaching a course on American literature. Why would anyone not rush to such a rare opportunity?)

I learned to write philosophy as the philosophers did and published in many of the most prestigious journals. Five years later my relationship to the discipline had changed. What made the difference was my emerging interest in decision-making in medicine—an interest that some within the core of the profession saw as "rather journalistic," uttered as a philosopher's term of denigration. Getting a grant to support that work gave it an aura of respectability in certain philosophical eyes and an odor of pandering to the market in certain philosophical noses. But the old idea of philosophy as an approach to understanding other domains had survived my transition into the profession and provided a bonus at that. In turning to the world of medicine and health care as a philosopher, I was brought back to some of those big questions that motivate so much early philosophical interest on the part of undergraduates, but which are understandably forced into the background in graduate programs that give pride of place to rigor and a mastery of the current literature in pure philosophy.

In thinking about medical care, one thinks about human frailty and mortality, about what in life is most valuable, about relationships of trust and caring. In asking how decisions in health policy should be made, one asks traditional questions of political philosophy about the fabric of social organization—about such matters as collective responsibility and individual liberty—but one asks them in a context of heightened intensity, since the health and even the lives of one's fellow humans may be influenced by how one answers.

Here, once again, a tension emerges, between the temptation to be of use—to bring one's philosophical and perhaps even rhetorical skills to bear on specific pending questions, and the imperative one was expected to internalize as a student philosopher to follow one's question tenaciously wherever it leads, without regard to practical matters or how much time it takes.

I realize that some of what I have done invites the observation that I have gone into philosophy and out the other side. Perhaps so, at least from time to time. But I am no longer concerned with the boundaries of the discipline. Such insouciance may even be a mark of progress. I know, at least, that everything I do bears the stamp, if not the standards, of my mentors—and that how I have approached administrative questions as well as intellectual ones—is as it is because my field is philosophy.

Each of the following stories reflects the same theme in one way or another. This theme results from my thinking about experiences I have had in the context of how they relate to other experiences and to the underlying values of curiosity, justice, beauty, and knowledge that animate philosophy in the first place. Each is a true story of how something I consider important looks to me now, beyond boundaries, approaching from above.

REFRAMING

"When we change the story and how we tell it, we can change the world."

—FrameWorks website, 2023

In 1975 the National Science Foundation and National Endowment for the Humanities jointly funded a *Summer Institute on Philosophical Ethics for Science and Engineering Faculty.* As Director, I chose Stanford as the venue. The forty faculty participants had comfortable on-campus housing at Escondido Village, family members had an ample array of appealing activities, and there were abundant recreational opportunities for participants seeking relief from the intense workload. Despite the Institute's name, my goal was for all participants to understand that science, engineering, and ethics are inextricably connected. They are not independent domains, each useful to know. They are bound together inseparably. So instead of teaching ethics to the scientists and engineers, my objective was to induce everyone to develop an integrated awareness of these domains. That reframing of the goal guided me in developing the program.

Cognitive scientists have long known that how an issue is framed can determine reactions to it. That knowledge guides much of what pollsters, advertisers, politicians, and even parents do. Yet, in moments of distress, it's easy to forget that reframing can solve a problem, as it did at the Institute. The presentations were made by some of us there for the duration plus a cascade of luminaries brought in for short intervals, including—Kenneth Arrow (Nobel Laureate in economics), Carl Hempel (who had participated in philosophy's legendary Vienna Circle in the 1940s), and Howard Raiffa (leading theoretician of decision analysis). Among the most lustrous was Eugene Wigner, who had won a Nobel Prize for theoretical work on particle physics. We all looked forward with eager anticipation to hearing him. But moments before he was to begin, as we were finishing lunch, he turned toward me and softly said, "I'm sorry. I can't do this. I just can't do it."

Shocked, I asked what the problem was. I worried that we needed an ambulance. He replied sadly, "If I talk about the physics, which the scientists and engineers mostly know, to avoid boring them I'll have to make it so technical the humanities faculty will be lost. If I make it understandable to the humanities people, the others will be completely bored. I will either be boring to half of them or incomprehensible to half of them. Either way, half will be disappointed, and this will be a failure. I can't do it."

I said, "I understand. You are right, and I can't ask you to do that. However, the science and engineering people, no matter how much physics they know, have never seen you explain that physics to a humanities audience. If you discuss the physics in a way the humanities people can understand, seeing how *you* do that will be new—and tremendously valuable—to the scientists and engineers. It will be a master class in the effective communication of science, something they all need to be able to do." After a brief, thoughtful look, he smiled broadly, nodded, and said, "I can do *that!*" With his task reframed, he went on and was brilliant.

I've often thought of that moment as a reminder when confronting some unexpected obstruction or sensing a teachable moment. A student asked, "What is your favorite color?" Rather than giving a facile response, I replied, "Why assume I have a favorite color? Favorite for *what*—? For a car, for a bedroom wall, for soup? These superlative modifiers are perilous. Why not reframe the question and ask about my color preferences in a more sophisticated and open way? Why not ask, 'What are some of your preferences regarding colors?'"

Early in the covid pandemic, an article in the *New Yorker* mentioned work I had done on the allocation of scarce medical resources in tragic situations. That prompted a deluge of media inquiries, domestic and international, about who should get access to ventilators when not enough were available. Each time, I deflected and reframed the question, explaining that the allocation of ventilators is not the primary question; rather, one ought to ask what is needed in personnel and infrastructure to make reasoned decisions and optimal treatment possible. Some reporters understood and wrote articles or did video interviews accordingly. Others disappeared to find someone to offer them rules for ventilator allocation. So reframing doesn't always work. Like any other strategy for conceptual clarification, it can open the mind or close the door.

(3)

THE REAL THING

---

*Can you tell the difference between a $10,000 Chanel
bag and a $200 knockoff? Almost nobody can . . .*

——Amy X Wang, the *New York Times*, May 4, 2023

When and why does it matter to have a real object on display
in a museum, rather than some representation of it—whether
electronic or any other variety of facsimile?

The eminent Shakespeare scholar Stephen Greenblatt, in
his Pulitzer Prize-winning book *The Swerve*, writes that " . . .
art always penetrates the fissures in one's psychic life." How
we will be struck by a painting, a piece of music, or an object
in an exhibition will depend, unpredictably, on who we are
and what will trigger an emotional reaction that transcends
an intellectual engagement with that art. We can be completely startled by this phenomenon.

David O'Hara (*Chronicle of Higher Education*, 8/16/2013, B 20) described such a moment vividly, recounting his first viewing of *Guernica*:

> I had no idea. This museum apparently was not a locked space for storing images; it was a classroom in which I could watch Picasso labor over this painting. . . . I took a breath, and walked briskly into the room, intending to keep my jaw firm, my spine straight, my knees steady. I turned and looked.
>
> And then I fell down . . .
>
> When I turned that corner and saw *Guernica* I had the feeling I was standing in front of something holy. . . . Picasso knocked me to my knees . . .

When I read that en route to Los Angeles to visit the Page Museum at the La Brea Tar Pits in August 2013, I knew what O'Hara meant. (More about that visit later.) Years earlier, I had seen the Darwin exhibition at the American Museum of Natural History. Although no expert, I knew about Darwin and his work. I'd read biographies, traced his steps in the Galapagos, extolled the literary virtues of his *Voyage of The Beagle*, seen the Darwin exhibition in London. Little in the AMNH exhibition was new to me. Then, suddenly, I was inches away from his magnifying glass—not a replica, but the real thing. He had held it, peered through it at specimens, relied on it in his monumental, tenacious effort to figure out how things work. And to my amazement, I had the feeling that I was standing in front of something holy.

Had the magnifying glass been a flawless facsimile—indistinguishable from the original but not misrepresented—it might have been worth seeing. But that sense of proximity to Darwin would have been missing. It was crucial that this was the real thing, although sometimes a facsimile is fine. What makes this difference?

Writing about art forger Mark Landis (*New Yorker*, August 26, 2013), Alec Wilkinson said:

> He believes that if something is beautiful, it doesn't matter whether it is genuine; rather, the impression it engenders is what counts. He thinks that he has given work to small museums that couldn't afford it, so that people who wouldn't usually encounter such pieces can see them and be broadened. This attitude accords with the earlier philosophies of American museums, which often presented facsimiles of European sculpture in the form of plaster casts. At one point the Museum of Fine Art in Boston had the third-largest collection of plaster casts in the world. "Initially there wasn't the mission among our museums that you needed to have original works of art," Henry Adams [professor of art at Case Western Reserve] told me.

Yet what counted for me in seeing Darwin's magnifying glass was not that he used one exactly *like* this, but that he had used *this*. The power of the perception depended on the provenance of the object, not on its observable physical properties.

Anne Fadiman, in "Marrying Libraries" (Chapter One of *Ex Libris*, a book I've savored at least a dozen times), addresses such issues, recalling how she and her husband chose which copies of books to keep. (If an unmarked copy was a gift from the author, does that have more value than an identical copy I had bought?)

Seeing the real thing can matter for reasons of scale and context. Whatever one has read, seen in photographs, or experienced in IMAX-scale documentaries, nothing approximates the impact of the golden dome in Jerusalem reflecting the magical light of the setting sun. Standing beneath the massive temple at Abu Simbel conveys a sense of scale and grandeur for which there can be no facsimile. (This is true, also, for natural wonders: the Grand Canyon can be seen only at the Grand Canyon; the falls at Iguazu, seen and heard and felt through the mist, can have no replica.)

Sometimes, what matters about the thing itself has to do with specificity of place. Walking among the ruins in Athens, one recalls the ancient thinkers who walked *here*, breathed this air under this sky. When I looked into the cell on Robben Island that held Mandela for so many years, my hands gripping the bars that constrained him, it was not just a sense of his history that gave the moment such impact. It was a sense of place—of seeing, and being, precisely where he had been.

Museums sometimes provide such encounters with immovable sights and sites when they sponsor trips, typically with docents—although too often a lockstep pace denies anyone the freedom to linger, reflect, and enter these portals to reverie. Immovable objects can be seen only in situ—be they works of architecture (Frank Gehry's Guggenheim-Bilbao, seen from the nearby bridge, arises like a great, gleaming flower above the multicolored boxcars in the railroad yard) or the Diego Rivera frescoes in the Detroit Institute of Art. The only option is to go to them.

Other artistically important objects can be moved only at great cost in money, time, and effort. The bronze doors by Ghiberti from the Battistero di San Giovanni in Florence—called *The Gates of Paradise* by Michelangelo and 21 years in the making—are among the glories of Florence. My Syracuse colleague Gary Radke spent five years collaborating with the High Museum of Atlanta, arranging to bring them to the United States following their restoration. I'd marveled at them in Florence, but seeing them in Seattle, viewing them closely from front and back, provided a sense of intimacy that was an enduring privilege. The renovated halls of Islamic Art at the Metropolitan Museum also exemplify this, with entire rooms transported from their original locations. So the distinction between movable and immovable objects is somewhat fluid. Sometimes the mountain does come to Mohammed.

In principle, even Rembrandt's *Night Watch* could travel. But when renowned treasures travel, viewers often wait in crowded lines for measured glimpses—as I once waited in London for four hours to see Tutankhamun's mask. *Seeing the Night Watch* means lingering before it, searching for the sources of light within it, attending to the shadows, the clothing, the markers of status or station—looking at it and into it over and over again, slowly. This is what was possible when the Pace Gallery gathered a large array of Rothko paintings at its former Soho location and allowed viewers to savor the paintings over extended time, as they changed and as the viewer's introspections evolved as well. That's rarely how we get to see the real thing when it comes to visit.

And as Radke explains, even when we visit an artistic venue in place, its context has changed over time. He notes:

" . . . the light and the surface condition . . . will usually have aged to something unrecognizable to original viewers." Regarding *The Gates of Paradise*, he adds, "Intimate viewing is the primary experience . . . but so is the sense of seeing 'the forbidden,' what in this case the artist hid behind the reliefs and never intended us to see."

Setting aside such outlier situations, we can clarify when the real thing matters essentially. It is when the viewer's knowledge (that the object in view is authentic) induces an emotional response to that fact: a sense of immediacy and connection that the object has the power to prompt precisely because it connects its history with that part of our own history.

MIT Professor Nancy Hopkins sought more office space but was denied repeatedly. She then investigated how much space different people had and documented her finding that male scientists were supported far more generously than female scientists. Her results catalyzed corrective measures at MIT and nationally. It's unfinished business, to be sure. But the story, told in the MIT Museum's EXHIBITION150, is represented by one iconic object: the modest tape measure Hopkins used in documenting the inequities. Any tape measure can measure an office or lab. Only *this* one is the one she used, and therein lies its special impact—its ability, in light of all it represents, to electrify the normally calm, accomplished, well-established scientist. (The full story of Hopkins' monumental achievement is told in Kate Zernike's compelling and comprehensive account, *The Exceptions: Nancy Hopkins, MIT, and the Fight for Women in Science*, 2023.)

At the Page Museum, almost everything is local and real. There's a diorama or two, but the millions of fossils on display and in storage were all found there at La Brea. A toe bone from a Paleolithic mouse may intrigue or amuse, but looking up at the tusks of the herbivorous woolly mammoth or at skeletons of carnivorous megafauna that once were looking for lunch right here inspires awe, much as the 5-foot-long head of Sue, the Field Museum's *Tyrannosaurus rex* does. If these were replicas, there could always be some small uncertainty (or comfort) in wondering whether the *real* thing is quite so scary. And the knowledge that one is seeing a replica intrudes a layer of distance between the viewer and the history of the object. A replica of the head of Sue had no ferocious roar, did not terrify prey, did not die in circumstances we would love to understand but will never know.

So it is with documents. In September 2012, huge crowds waited in Syracuse to see Lincoln's handwritten preliminary Emancipation Proclamation from September 1862. Reluctant to turn viewers away, an exhausted staff voluntarily stayed on for hours after the official closing time of the exhibition, aware of the emotional power of an encounter between a viewer and the hand of Lincoln—not the equal of shaking his massive, world-changing hand, but as close to that as we can get. A replica could have the same text and appearance. It could not have the same emotional power.

An especially memorable example of this point followed Elie Wiesel's visit to our campus. He was one of the few people I have ever seen receive a standing ovation the instant he appeared on stage. During his visit I had the privilege of spending time with him, including a quiet and unhurried breakfast, just three people, prior to his departure. Shortly thereafter, I visited the Holocaust Museum in Washington. I had his short, overwhelming book *Night* well in mind as I entered the crowded museum. Among the objects on display was a boxcar. Not a replica—a boxcar used to transport Jews, and of course many others, to extermination camps. A ramp led to the open boxcar door. I paused there, as the content of

Night flashed through my mind. Then I slowly entered. No one else was in the boxcar. Despite the crowd in the museum, I was suddenly alone. I stood there hearing the sounds that Elie had described so vividly. I felt the heat, imagined the stench, the fear, the despair. I thought of those who suffered in this boxcar, not a boxcar like this, but *this one*. I also thought of the holds of the *Isabella* and the *Amistad*. When I left through the other side, I could not read the wall signs through my tears.

Today, we struggle to dismantle 400-year-old structures of racism and to acknowledge the pervasive white privilege that sustains them. We know that discomfort is unavoidable. We all have boxcars we don't want to enter. Terrible recent events have helped shine a light on those boxcars and confirm that they are the real thing. We must do all we can to destroy the structures that make them possible.

Sometimes what we seek in looking at an artifact, a fossil, or a document is just information, be it a text, structure, or design. A facsimile then can serve us well. But the stakes are higher, the purposes deeper, when we want a sense of immediacy and personal connection with an important part of our own past or of the world we want to understand much better. Whether we are emotionally open to that depends on us. But when we are, that's when only the real thing will do.

VALUES, CAUSATION, THEISM, AND THE MORAL COMMUNITY

I want to respond to the view of secular humanism. But I find it difficult to explode a bomb and get away in two minutes.

—Hassan Hathout (1984)

VOULIAGMENI, 1984

In the beautiful resort of Vouliagmeni, by the Aegean Sea, I gave an address about life, suffering, and death from the stage of a packed conference hall. My task, assigned by the conference organizers Zbigniew Bankowski and John Bryant, was to discuss those topics from the perspective of secular humanism. That is what I did. My colleague Ed Pellegrino, a physician and president of The Catholic University of America, was asked to present a Christian perspective; in doing what he was assigned to do he carefully avoided presenting his own perspective as a Catholic. I concluded my presentation by saying:

> Secular humanism is a viewpoint that places human welfare at the center of the moral universe and looks empirically to the way the world works in order to determine what is right and what is wrong. It is a doctrine of reason, compassion, respect, charity, and tolerance, not because those values are divinely inspired but because those are the values that work best. In advocating them, it keeps company with much of what is central in many of the world's religious traditions, which, while they are not secular, are often humane.

When discussion opened, with a two-minute limit per speaker, Dr. Hassan Hathout spoke first. He decried the absence in my comments of any theologically grounded and inviolable standards of behavior and causally linked that absence to a wide array of what he considered disasters. He said:

> I want to respond to the view of secular humanism. But I find it difficult to explode a bomb and get away in two minutes.

> I do respect the different views and I think we are all for the ethics of disagreement, and I hope we keep up to the standard in this. However, I am puzzled, because when I look around myself I find Jews, Christians, and Muslims, and then I find a paper which was

not distributed beforehand that tells us not against Moses, but if he tells us that his commandments are God's values to guide our life, we should tell him get lost. Human values should originate from human beings.

Again, Jesus came with teachings and if He says these are God's teachings, we tell him, no, we don't believe you, get lost. Values of people should emanate from people, and the same with Muslims. If this is true, two things would follow.

The first, if I shared your beliefs, sir, was that upon the first suffering in my life, and my life includes many sufferings, I would have found it quite logical to go and take 100 sleeping pills and go to bed to sleep, never to be disturbed again.

The second thing, if what you say is true, then I would like to congratulate you for the epidemic of venereal disease, for the success of homosexuality as a movement, for the development of AIDS and other diseases, for man's exploitation of man throughout history, because this is the result of human values being derived from just human sources. With all due respect to your views, we believe that we were created by God and, whether you are against Him or not, if we believe in Him, we should believe that He gave us the values to live with and we live with these values in democracy, but under God. And, I think democracy falls into a great fallacy, because once you can summon enough of a majority to decree that there is no God, you will have it under a Godless, democratic system. I think that this is all I can say in two minutes.

The audience had gasped audibly at Hathout's first comment. Now the moderator, seeming startled and uncomfortable, hesitated, looked around, and asked if I would care to respond. I did:

Yes, I would welcome a moment to reply. I could use the rest of the conference, but I will restrict myself to a few brief points. I was asked to describe for this group the views of secular humanism and that is what I tried to do. I think I described them reasonably accurately. I said nothing about my own beliefs except in respect to the case of Mr. Bartling [explained below]. I have no apology for that position.

I will now say a bit more about my beliefs. One of my beliefs is that nothing that is said in a dialogue should inspire anyone to think of exploding a bomb. That is not the way to resolve differences of opinion. Nothing that I said, I think, should have induced anyone to think that a secular humanist response to the claims of Moses or Jesus or Mohammed or anyone else is "get lost." Rather, the response is more likely to be "I respect those values too, though I have a different opinion about where they came from." That is what much of the point of my paper was designed to show.

Also, I am quite surprised that the inference of anything I said suggested ready recourse to suicide as the analgesic of first resort. On the contrary, I think that it is a part of human secular (the secular humanist) approach to struggle very vigorously to maximize human well-being, and that includes helping people with physical and psychological problems to circumvent those problems.

I suppose there is a certain pride that one could take in being accused all at once of venereal disease throughout the world, homosexuality, AIDS, and much of the rest of (what you consider) the evils that beset mankind, but all I can say about those accusations as an inference on the content of my remarks is that it is an impressive exercise in creative listening. And I'll say nothing more.[1,2]

More than 200 people rose in an immediate standing ovation. A dozen or so remained seated—motionless, silent. When the session ended and I descended from the stage, a well-dressed man approached, extended his hand, and introduced himself as a physician from Turkey. He was among those I had noticed sitting silent and expressionless during the outburst of support for my rejoinder. He said, "I am a Muslim and a believer. But I tell you that there is no place in civilized discourse or in Islam for such comments as were made to you, and I repudiate them." I thanked him warmly but felt tremendous sadness that he had not felt free to express his dissenting view openly.

This story is not merely about my personal history. It's a case study in how we attribute causation, how we assess personal character, how we define a moral community with or without theism, and how we see beyond the boundaries of our own perspectives, especially in morally charged situations.

THE CAUSAL CHAIN

There in Vouliagmeni, unbeknownst to me, was Spyros Doxiadis, the Greek Minister of Health. That evening he phoned with an invitation to dinner, beginning a relationship that quickly led to collaborative work. The conference had been sponsored by CIOMS—the Council of International Organizations of Medical Sciences—an NGO (Non-Governmental Organization) affiliated with and located at the World Health Organization (WHO). Almost every year CIOMS held a meeting somewhere. Following the episode in Vouliagmeni, I was invited to one CIOMS event after another—in Ixtapa, Mexico; in Bangkok, Thailand; in Noordwijk aan Zee, the Netherlands; and often at WHO in Geneva. Dr. Alfred Gellhorn, an officer of CIOMS, had also been at Vouliagmeni. An elegant and patrician physician of great distinction, he, too, was at these subsequent events. I quickly came to admire, and enjoy working with, him.

In August 1986, I became dean of the college of arts and sciences at Syracuse University. The former dean had becomec vice-chancellor for academic affairs—and thus my new boss. He had clear ideas about what a dean should and should not do, and it did not take long for him to have misgivings about the appointment he had just made. A chemist, he'd abandoned both research and teaching when he became an administrator. He wanted me to do the same: to accept my new role as a pure manager.[3] Over his explicit objections, I continued to publish at least a small amount each year and to teach one course every year—except for the year I cancelled my course because of the destruction, in December 1988, of PanAm Flight 103. Thirty-five of our students perished, along with hundreds of others, including eleven citizens of Lockerbie incinerated in their homes. Someone had indeed exploded a bomb at them.

Having dealt with the immediate aftermath of that murderous event, I recoil at talk of exploding bombs at people. When I stood by the memorial *bothy*—a small rural shelter beside the Tundergarth church near Lockerbie, where I had placed a wreath on behalf of my university—a somber young man approached, thanked me, pointed to a sloping field nearby, and said, "That's where they found my brother's body." I would have liked to turn then to Dr. Hathout and ask him, "Is this what you had in mind?"

Also in 1988 I received a call from David Axelrod, Commissioner of Health for New York State. To my amazement, he conveyed a request from Governor Mario Cuomo that I accept appointment to an advisory body the governor had created in 1985 by Executive Order: the New York State Task Force on Life and the Law. This group of two dozen people was charged to assist the state in developing policies on issues at the interface of medicine, law, and ethics. It was a compelling and flattering invitation, but I knew better than to accept. I told Dr. Axelrod I had to check with my boss and asked for a couple of days. The VCAA's immediate response was unequivocal: *No.* He said it would distract from my responsibilities without compensatory benefits for the university and was not acceptable. I reported that, sadly, to Dr. Axelrod. Then *he* asked for a couple of days.

About two days later the vice-chancellor called and said he had been thinking it over, that he could see some benefits for the University after all—in cooperating with the state and in public service—and that he'd changed his mind and thought I should accept. I called Axelrod and thanked him for what I assumed was a persuasive call to my boss. "Oh, no," he replied. "I did not call him." Instead, he revealed, he had called the chancellor to say that the governor had a complaint about one of the faculty, who had mysteriously declined the governor's request for assistance. The chancellor then told the vice-chancellor there was a problem with Gorovitz that he'd better straighten out quickly. I told Axelrod I had never seen such brilliant political maneuvering, but I did not tell the vice-chancellor that I knew the real story behind his duplicitous "rethinking."

I had no idea what led to Governor Cuomo's request. Only later did I learn that the principal health policy advisor to Commissioner Axelrod was Alfred Gellhorn, then director of medical affairs for the New York State Department of Health. He had admired what he heard in Vouliagmeni and enjoyed our collaborations at later CIOMS events, and he had rec-ommended me for the Task Force. So I joined the Task Force in 1988 and have been on it ever since. We've done reports on many subjects: Physician Assisted Suicide, Surrogate Decision-making, Assisted Reproductive Technologies, and many more. It has been an opportunity to do hard, serious work on challenging problems with impressive and dedi-cated colleagues.

The Task Force is chaired by the commissioner, and David Axelrod was deeply involved in our work. His incapacitating stroke in 1991 and premature death in 1994 dealt a tremen-dous blow to public health in New York. His successors as commissioner have spanned the gamut from the indifferent, to the felonious, to the superb. None more clearly exemplified the superb than Dr. Richard F. Daines, whose sudden death in February 2011 was also an incalculable loss.

I was delighted that Alfred Gellhorn had an office exactly where the Task Force met. Often, I would visit him. We collaborated on further CIOMS projects, chatted about Task Force topics, and even talked about how he might best help Caroline Moorehead, the British biographer of his late sister Martha Gellhorn, a legendary war correspondent who had briefly been married to Ernest Hemingway. Alfred had many letters from Martha, copies of which he sent to Moorehead. Having often visited Martha in London, he had many English friends and colleagues. When he died at 94 in 2008, Cynthia Kee, in *The Guardian*, noted that he had "infused medical education with a sense of social mission, bringing in women and minorities." Gellhorn had been the ideal medical advisor for a commissioner who sought to advance social justice through the mechanisms of government.

The Task Force's work on genetic testing and screening brought us into close association with New York's highly distinguished Wadsworth Laboratory. When New York State established a stem cell initiative and legislatively mandated the process by which its board would be created, the governor's office turned for advice to senior staff within the Department of Health. Administrative responsibility for the venture was lodged in the Wadsworth Laboratory, and Larry Sturman was named executive director of NYSTEM—the research initiative to be overseen by the board. Immersed in my university work, I knew nothing of these events. In June 2007, I received puzzling messages about some state committee request, and assumed these were Task Force related. Once I learned they were about a new Stem Cell Board, I quickly looked into this. I discovered that Sturman, and other advisors, had proposed my appointment primarily because of their familiarity with work I had done for the Task Force—which I would not have been on but for Hathout and the episode in Vouliagmeni. Shortly before his spectacular self-destruction as governor, Eliot Spitzer appointed me to the Empire State Stem Cell Board, created to oversee a $600 million investment in stem cell research.

CAUSATION, RELIGION, MORALITY

The issues raised by that episode are both ancient and current. Socrates, in Plato's dialogue *The Euthyphro*, argued powerfully that morality cannot logically be based on religion. That kind of talk led to his death by hemlock. The Scottish philosopher David Hume developed the same position far more extensively (many would say *definitively*), in his *Dialogues Concerning Natural Religion*, but he had the prudence to publish it posthumously. Senator Joseph Lieberman, without the bomb talk, sides with Dr. Hathout. Lieberman has claimed that "the Constitution guarantees freedom of religion, not freedom from religion," adding, "George Washington warned us never to indulge the supposition that morality can be maintained without religion."

The Necessity Claim—that morality *requires* religion—is ambiguous. It can mean (Necessity Claim One) that as a matter of human *psychology* people will behave ethically only if motivated by religious reasons. Or it can mean (Necessity Claim Two) that as a matter of *logic*, only religious reasons can justify moral conclusions. Both claims are common, but neither has been conclusively defended. That is why the secular humanist position deserved inclusion at the conference, despite Dr. Hathout's diatribe, and why it deserves still to be a respected point of view despite the frantic rantings of people like the fundamentalist ideologue and political opportunist Michelle Bachmann, who endorsed the claim that "'The Secular Humanist Worldview' is one of America's greatest threats." And she later suggested that earthquakes and hurricanes, such as Irene, are divine retribution for our considering increasing some government revenue streams. Her backpedaling campaign apologists then said we should not take her statement seriously. In contrast, James Wood, a rational thinker, pointed out in a *New Yorker* article that secular humanism can be "as attuned to human need as religion has been, and as responsive to social injustice as the teachings of Jesus or Muhammad."[4]

Hathout's blast had not come from some rough-hewn radical firebrand. He was an Egyptian-born physician with doctoral degrees from both Cairo and Edinburgh, who had practiced medicine for twenty-six years (and co-founded a medical school) in Kuwait before moving to California in the 1980s. He had heroically saved wounded Jewish soldiers during the Siege of Ramle, when Israeli forces invaded a Palestinian village in one of the bloodiest episodes of the 1948 war. Later, he was a leading advocate of tolerant inter-faith dialogue, working effectively with Christian and Jewish leaders to establish bridge-building programs. He called on Muslims to spurn anti-American rhetoric, and on everyone to cease classifying people by religion. He saw himself as being, and called on others to be, motivated by "a loving heart." His death at 84 in 2009 was widely mourned by religious leaders of many faiths. And yet, this highly educated, cultivated, accomplished, courageous, scholarly, and gentle professional had invoked the notion of bomb-throwing as his immediate response to me. His loving heart did not extend to those he saw as lacking commitment to a religious tradition as the only possible foundation for morality.

Hathout's brief statement is rich with puzzling causal conjectures. He identifies what he considers undesirable phenomena (some actually so, such as "man's exploitation of man"), and makes clear that secular humanism is fundamentally unacceptable to his perspective. If the secular humanists were right, he says, their beliefs would be the cause of the phenomena he laments. He gives no hint of how that causation could possibly work. But he rejects secular humanism as false, so it isn't the cause of all those sorrows, after all. He seems untroubled by the obvious remaining question: what then *is* the cause of these alleged calamities? That's the classic "problem of evil" which every theistic position must address.

These causal conjectures are his garbled way of affirming both versions of the Necessity Claim: that without religion, there is no logical basis for requiring morality and there is no motivation to be virtuous. Those who do not embrace religion are therefore apparently outside the moral community. He seems entirely unaware of this simple and powerful challenge to the Necessity Claims: *In the absence of basic human decency, religious conviction is not sufficient to cause virtuous behavior, and in the presence of basic human decency, religious conviction is not needed to cause virtuous behavior.*

OPEN AND SHUT

In both the Task Force and the Stem Cell Board, we always sought and deeply respected the many voices of religious traditions. We also wrestled with the perennial question of what influence religious perspectives should have on public policy and on spending public funds in ethically contested domains. Task Force meetings are closed; its members are forbidden to disclose any content from those meetings to non-members. When we finish a project, we issue a report. No one can learn what we say among ourselves. Stem Cell Board meetings, however, were legislatively required to be transparent: open to the public and webcast in real time. (That board, its funds fully expended, is no longer active.)

Anyone with internet access, anywhere, could hear what we said as we said it, or later via an archived copy of the webcast. We were even forbidden to discuss any board business with one another outside the open meetings. There are reasons for this difference. The Task Force was created by, and as advisory to, the Executive Branch; the Stem Cell Board was created by, and constrained by, statute. But the juxtaposition makes salient the question of what sorts of business are best conducted openly and what sorts in private. In countless domains—the physician's office, the lawyer's conference, the patent application meeting, the religious confessional, the football huddle, and many more—we vigorously defend the sanctity of the secret.

In Task Force meetings, with intense mutual respect, members negotiate positions with candor and courage— changing their minds in response to better arguments, trying out controversial positions, brainstorming creatively. I heard clergy of a single denomination and of different denominations strategizing about how to frame arguments that would avoid opposition by reactionary authorities within their own religious organizations. Such candid exchanges among trusting colleagues facilitate progress and effective resolution but cannot happen before video cameras. Transparency can be repressive. The Turkish physician who approached me required privacy to express his dissent from Hathout's inflammatory rhetoric. And I doubt Hathout would have spoken so easily of exploding a bomb had he been on camera before the world. Yet secrecy can be toxic, as we too often discover.

In Plato's *Republic*, Claucon tells of a magic ring that can make its wearer invisible, and claims that "no man can be imagined to be of such an iron nature that he would stand fast in justice" given such a ring. Secrecy is a way of keeping things invisible, and when those in power decide what is to be secret (or, in current terms, classified as Top Secret), the potential for abuse of power is immense. The results can include loss of assets, violation of basic rights, deprivation of liberty, and even loss of life. Decent authorities, of course, will have no part in such unethical and even vile doings. But bad actors abound in high places, as well as in low, and a cloak of darkness is their ally. If fear of divine retribution does not deter them, the loss of secrecy might.

It is often hard to find or fashion a viable balance between transparency and confidentiality. There's no algorithm for that, no set of procedures that will lead directly to the best result. Good judgment and good character are essential. So are processes of review and accountability, with quality control mechanisms that resist corruption. What works for personal medical records won't be what protects intellectual property rights; what secures a journalist's sources won't be quite right for effective international diplomacy. What works for one religious leader may fail for another. Tensions among competing values—such as secrecy and transparency, or many others—typically lead to unstable resolution. When one value is favored, it generates oppositional pressures in support of the less favored values.

In Task Force and Stem Cell Board meetings, I some-times paused to be sure about whether I was in the secret conversation or the transparent one. In both, we strove—but in different ways—to understand what actions are likely to cause what effects on the well-being of individual people and on populations. Often, this leads to examining what has happened, and to inquire about the causal history of the events and situations that interest us. The answers are rarely clear, rarely easy. The cause of illness in a patient and the epi-demiology of disease in a population are the stuff of detec-tives, of hypothesis-conjurers, of sleuths who work to prove themselves wrong as they try to get closer to what might be true. They must constantly ask the fundamental epistemological questions: what do we think we know and why do we think we know it? They are part medical folks, part Sherlock Holmes, part David Hume.

CAUSATION AND CHARACTER

Hume worried about our ability to make sense of causation, noting that all judgments about cause and effect rely on past experience—but we can never be sure that the future will conform to the past. It doesn't help to claim that so far it always has. And even when we are sure that one kind of event is regularly associated with another, we risk mistaking constant conjunction for causal connection. Claims about causation are exceedingly difficult to confirm, and Hume was skeptical about our ability ever to do so. He saw causal judgment as an epistemological quagmire.

My father's father, Benjamin Gorovitz, came here from the town of Kreslava in the province of Vitebsk (then in Latvia) in 1908 to escape military conscription and other oppressions. Born Eingoren, on arrival he adopted the name of his older half-brother Aaron Gorovitz who was already here and served as his sponsor. As one biographer put it, Aaron, who came to be known as "the Dean of the Orthodox Rabbinate in greater Boston," was "distinguished as a pioneer for his efforts and achievements in building and nurturing the greater Boston Jewish community in the first half of [the twentieth] century. He was known for trying to 'strengthen Judaism from within and to build a bridge of understanding between the Jews and Christians in the community,' at a time when most others avoided this type of outreach."[5]

Benjamin, too, had been trained as a rabbi, and quickly obtained a rabbinical license in Bristol, Rhode Island, on

September 4 of that year. He even had a small congregation briefly in Attleboro, Massachusetts. But that was not viable, and he moved to Hyde Park, Massachusetts, where he found work in the kosher meat business. In the 1920s, this poor and pious man bought a cigarette–rolling machine; it was less costly to roll one's own. Then he read a report from the Metropolitan Life Insurance Co. that smokers had higher rates of various diseases. To undermine one's health was a sin, so he just quit smoking. I admire that. But his new machine was going to waste, and waste was a sin. He thought of giving it to a friend, but to undermine the health of another was also a sin. What then was he to do?

There seemed no solution. I picture him at the kitchen table, anxiously poring over the *Talmud* for guidance. But then he found his way. A Christian man worked at the synagogue on the Sabbath; the machine went to him. I do *not* admire *that*. Apparently that worker was outside the relevant moral community. How I wish I could orchestrate a conversation between the devout Hathout and my devout grandfather about who counts for what, and why. (If Hathout was right, perhaps they're debating it now, with Uncle Aaron as moderator.)

But as uncertain as he was about the machine, my grandfather had no uncertainty about smoking. The correlation was enough for him. There was no general understanding then of the causal connection between smoking and illness, and the industry deftly exploited that fact for more than half a century. Perhaps some third factor caused people to smoke and also to become ill. Perhaps illness caused people to seek comfort in smoking. Perhaps it was coincidence. Only slowly did the links in the causal chain emerge, as the processes of toxicity became known at the molecular level.

Once the industry was forced, over its strong objections, to print warnings about the health effects of tobacco, it sought refuge in the claim that the cause of tobacco-related illness was the smoker's culpable disregard for those explicit warnings. But the industry knew more than it let on about the addictive nature of nicotine. It had used that knowledge to secure future markets by inducing children to develop the addiction that would kill so many of them later (while yielding great profits for the industry). Industry leaders had lied to the public and even to Congress. (In 2009, the U.S. Court of Appeals for the District of Columbia found that "we are not dealing with accidental falsehoods, or sincere attempts to persuade; Defendants' liability rests on deceits perpetrated with knowledge of their falsity.") The whole saga, beginning to end, was about the attribution of causation as a means of shaping judgments about responsibility. The industry, attributing causation to the smoker's actions, hoped to avoid being seen as a causal agent itself. They were using causal attribution as a way to advance their own interests.

Consider, too, a claim that HIV-AIDS is caused by a virus that should be combated by medical or pharmacological means, and a counterclaim that it is caused by inappropriate behavior—of a sort that the suitably devout or the truly moral or the rationally careful would always avoid. That's a Hathoutian claim. Naming a cause is often *not* an objective assessment of a purely factual matter. It reflects a prior sense of what values are preferred, what behavior is favored, what interests are at stake, what modes of intervention are most easily available, and what actions are most likely to cause desired outcomes.

The British philosopher R. G. Collingwood gave a classic example of this aspect of causal attribution in 1940, discussing an automobile accident on a dangerous road. The highway engineer attributes the accident to faulty banking of the curving road as compared with standards of the profession; others see the cause as the driver's imprudent speed or flaws in the design of the vehicle. Each of these causal attributions reflects a different judgment about what factors could have been influenced by whom, and about what behavior is culpable: Who had a responsibility to have acted differently in the long chain of events culminating in the crash? Insurance companies, litigators, and law enforcement authorities can look for the facts about terms of coverage, legal obligations, and formalized responsibilities as foundations for their reactions to the accident. But judgments about causal responsibility transcend formal obligations. They reflect a broader sense of who ought to have done what. They are value-based claims.

If we had an infallible algorithm to identify culpable action, we might ascribe causal responsibility more confidently. The quest for such moral certainty is exemplified by Hathout's insistence on divine values, immune to the vicissitudes of human sentiments and protected against the excesses of democracy. But the case for a divine origin of moral directives requires first being able to make clear sense of talk about divine things. If nothing literally divine is real, then moral directives cannot have divine origins. Speaking of the divine would then be either embracing an illusion or speaking metaphorically, inviting contested interpretations.

Advocates of Necessity Claim One (that moral *motivation* requires religion), having made a point about human psychology, are challenged by the evidence. They need no recourse to theology; they claim only that people must believe in divine directives to be motivated to do what is right. It should not matter whether those beliefs are actually true. Since Aristotle, however, the literature of moral psychology, and its successors in cognitive psychology and even neuroscience, have shown that virtuous action need not be motivated by religious reasons. It can be, and often is. But it need not be.

Advocates of Necessity Claim Two (that moral *justification* requires religion) commonly seek to ground their view that morality logically requires religion in a prior proof that only a divine cause can explain the existence of the visible universe. Once having secured that foundation, they then draw moral conclusions from it. Hume rejected every argument in favor of a divine creator, one by one, pointing out that the phenomena of our experience are compatible with so many different and conflicting hypotheses that there can be no rational basis for favoring any one over any other. Ever the empiricist, he held that all knowledge about the world must be based on experience of—and thus necessarily within—the world. He cautioned, "Our experience, so imperfect in itself and so limited both in extent and duration, can afford us no probable conjecture concerning the whole of things." He considered all causal conjecture about the origin of the universe to be unintelligible.

And Hume *severed* the linkage between religion and morality. He argued that only human sentiments can motivate our actions and that allegedly divine directives either are too obscure to be useful or are impossible to defend, except on grounds which have no reliance on religious claims. His view of moral directives is explicit:—they can and do arise only from human sentiment. What we value—and only that—accounts for what is valuable. Almost two centuries later, Collingwood *strengthened* the linkage between what we value and how we use causal language; he helped us understand that what we claim did happen, and what we claim does happen, are influenced by what we value and our beliefs about what should happen.

Sometimes, in making a causal claim, we are using our best critical skills to understand the processes of the physical world. That's what happened when John Snow found that contaminated water was causing the cholera epidemic in London in 1854. His inquiry was factual and scientific; his causal analysis led to major public health benefits as the old "miasma" theory of disease gave way to an empirically grounded epidemiology. This is the mission of science: to formulate hypotheses about how the world works and put them to the test of encounters with the evidence, by seeking to falsify them. But gathering, describing, and assessing evidence are each extremely hard. Further, even careful scientists are prone to confirmation bias (the tendency to see what they are looking for and to favor evidence that supports the hypotheses they favor). So skepticism about causal judgments, especially about one's own, is a requirement of intellectual integrity.

COMPLEXITIES OF CAUSAL JUDGMENT

That inherent difficulty of scientific inquiry is the first complexity of causal attribution. The second is the interconnectedness of the many causal chains that blend into the narrative that is the backstory of any important event. I emphasized the importance of the episode at Vouliagmeni in telling the story of how I came to be on the Stem Cell Board. But Alfred Gellhorn's appointment as medical advisor to the commissioner was also a necessary condition of my further adventures, as were the circumstances that moved me to New York State in 1986. Each of these factors, and countless others, has its own narrative. The way they merged and evolved is the full story of how I got to the board. In providing a causal narrative, the most we can ever do is select from among all the factors a few that seem to us, the storytellers, the most salient and best suited to our purposes. It can never be the full story. That's the second complexity.

The third complexity is that sometimes in making causal claims we are not so much seeking truth as lobbying for a preferred position about human behavior, expressing an opinion about what can best be influenced, or promoting a position about how responsibility should be assigned. This is the character of Hathout's causal claims, and of Senator Lieberman's, and of the tobacco industry flacks. It's a kind of causal assertion we see all around us, in politics, advertising, and even health-care policy debate. This is value judgment behind a veneer of ostensible factual objectivity. We advance our causes in part by the causal claims we make. We can't end that pervasive phenomenon, but we surely want to discern it—when others do it and, perhaps especially, if we do it ourselves. We want to see it for what it is and evaluate it with rigor and integrity.

CODA

On September 11, 2001, terrorists destroyed the World Trade Center. Most of us have vivid, detailed memories of the moment we learned of this—where we were, who was present, what we saw. And we trust those memories. Yet scientific studies of memory have proven that such memories—though clear, strong, and vivid— are highly inaccurate. We do not know as much as we think we know. We are well advised to be humble about our memories, our attitudes, and even our most confident convictions.

This much is indisputable: in that attack on the United States, about 3,000 people died initially. Thirty were Syracuse University alumni. Some politicians and even some journalists claimed the event killed nearly 3,000 Americans, and that claim persists in the media. I heard it on MSNBC in August 2022. Yet those who died came from many lands; 21 percent were born in other countries. Political rhetoric, and media coverage too, are often inaccurate. Recall the bombing in Oklahoma City in 1995. Many initial news stories blamed Islamic terrorists, such as those who masterminded the 1993 World Trade Center bombing. Some Americans responded to the Oklahoma bombing by attacking Muslims and people of Arab descent, even though the terrorists were Americans. This was triply wrong. First, Muslims had nothing to do with that bombing. Second, even if the terrorists had been Muslims, there is no justification for discriminating against other, uninvolved Muslims. Third, spontaneous vengeance is not a civilized way to respond even to the guilty.

Recall also Baruch Goldstein, the American-born, Jewish, Israeli physician who caused the Cave of the Patriarchs massacre in 1994 in Hebron, killing 29 Muslims at prayer and wounding 125. Would we agree that his terrorist actions show that Israelis or Jews in general are dangerous or deserve to be attacked? We know better, and we resent and resist efforts to stereotype anyone in any such way. The Israeli government condemned the massacre and arrested the other followers of the extremist Meir Kahane, forbidding certain settlers from entering Arab towns and demanding that those settlers turn in their rifles. Yet Goldstein's grave became a pilgrimage site for a few Jewish extremists. In 1999, after Israeli legislation outlawed monuments to terrorists, the Israeli army had to dismantle a shrine built to Goldstein.

Goldstein was properly denounced by mainstream Orthodox Judaism and widely considered insane by Israelis. He was a deranged individual, not part of an organization like Jihadist members of Al-Qaeda. His actions were tragic, but not part of something much larger and sustained. If we know a person is a part of Al-Qaeda, we have grounds to view him as an enemy on the basis on that affiliation. If we know only that he is a Muslim, or an Arab, we have no such grounds.

Daniel Barenboim, a musician of towering artistry and humanity, understood the folly of treating real people as stereotypes. He presented a free classical concert in Gaza City. The young people there, hearing Mozart rather than mortars, know from their own experience that Israelis can be decent, caring, fair-minded people—just as they know this also about most of their own brethren. And Nelson Mandela understood. He did not demonize the prison guards who oppressed him; he treated them with such respect that they ultimately became his students.

Yad Vashem may be the most powerfully moving place on earth. We should indeed never forget why it is there and what it means. Part of what we should never forget is that the evil that made Yad Vashem necessary was made easier by America's history of dehumanizing Blacks—a history of our own evil, publicly affirmed, reflected in our laws, cited explicitly by the Nazis, and defended even now by some Americans on grounds of their own religious or political convictions.

We have much to answer for in our treatment of Native Americans, Asian-Americans, our own Muslim population—a gentle and peace-loving people—and many other groups. We Americans are not an evil people, but we do evil when we judge anyone stereotypically and unthinkingly demonize those we see as different. Doing that is deeply embedded in the outlook of fundamentalists of all sorts—whether in a minaret or Mea Shearim. It's an outlook that leads extremists to explode bombs at people, to fly into office towers, to rip children from their families and send them off to extermination camps or reeducation centers that exterminate their cultural heritage, or to immigration-control cages that will traumatize them irreparably.

What happened at the World Trade Center was horrible. But what was most horrible is not just the many deaths. It is the toxic mindset that stereotypes, demonizes, and dehumanizes others—excluding them from the moral community for reasons that do not reflect their individual characters. That is wrong when it is done to any of us, and equally wrong when done *by* us. It was wrong of Hathout and wrong of my grandfather, both devout and fundamentally decent people, with a theistically based sense of the moral community that was too parochial.

This is not a new point, of course, and many people have been making it. Yet it is too easily and too often overlooked even by people who make it. We are all subject to the aforementioned confirmation bias—that powerful tendency to embrace evidence that supports what we prefer to believe and reject evidence that challenges what we think we know. The requirements of rigorous ethical inquiry, however, oblige us to seek evidence that can falsify our favored views—knowing that if we fail to find it, we will have stronger grounds for our beliefs. Doing that takes the courage to risk being wrong and, even worse, perhaps having to admit it and change our minds. Few of us always excel at such admissions.

I was horrified by Hassan Hathout's first words and all that they suggested. As I learned more about him, I came to have a deep appreciation of the complexity of his views and his character. I learned of his many virtues, including much greater respect for others than I initially realized he had. He also had an unwavering commitment to an exclusionary perspective I find intolerable. Yet I am a beneficiary of his intolerance. Had he not dismissed my comments so dramatically, and with such bizarre causal confusions, my comments would likely have been barely noticed, ephemeral remarks. I'm fortunate that he provided my launch toward great opportunities, and I wish I could have a leisurely conversation with him about all the ensuing events and the issues they prompt me to consider.

I'd like to send him a Thank You note—not an email or an electronic card with stylish visual images and professional music, but a *proper* note of appreciation, with my own words, handwritten carefully on a tasteful card. But it's too late. He's gone, and I don't have his forwarding address.

A PULITZER PRIZE

"Her English is too good," he said. "That clearly indicates that she is foreign."

—Zoltan Kaparthy in *My Fair Lady*,
played by Theodore Bikel (1964)

In the restaurant of the historic Pulitzer Hotel in Amsterdam, the server greeted me with an enthusiastic smile and some unintelligible words. I don't know Dutch, but I'd been hearing it each day and the server's language didn't sound like that. I asked if he spoke English; he beamed, nodded, and replied, "Little some try."

"Ah, good," I said, and asked for some water. He was bewildered. I lifted the empty water glass and repeated, "Water." "Yes, yes," he said. "You want with or without gasoline?" I was relieved to be in a non-smoking environment. "Thank you, with *gas* please," I replied. I learned later that he was from

Yugoslavia, recently arrived in Amsterdam, working hard to learn both Dutch and some English as he strove to better his prospects. That seemed impressively courageous.

One of the many respects in which America continues to be a great, albeit imperfect country, is evident whenever we consider going to a restaurant. We can choose among cuisines from all over the world, and in some areas from our indigenous cultures also. This array is a gift from our immigrant populations—which is almost all of us. It is a hallmark of our values that we welcome people from other lands, near or far. Because many of our immigrant communities are large enough to sustain a market for specialized ingredients, we can also cook at home, trying our hand at cuisines from every inhabited continent. This is possible only because our immigrant communities sustain these markets—which I have always found enthusiastically welcoming. Cuisine, of course, is always about much more than just food. It is about memory, politics, culture, relationships, and identity.

We hear much ignorant trash talk about immigrants, but not much about how they actually talk in restaurants. Many of the servers, in restaurants of all kinds, are learning English as they work. When I am greeted by the inappropriate, "How are we this evening," or asked, "Are we having wine tonight?" I want to scream, "Don't you even know the difference between *we* and *you*? Such banal blather is invariably inflicted on me by an "American," one whose first language, such as it is, is English. The recent immigrants are more careful, more concerned to get the language right, eager both to serve and to learn. They work hard and exude a sense of gratitude for the opportunity. They know what work is and do not shirk from it.

When a server looks at my plate and asks, "Are you still working on it?" I know it is more unthinking prattle by an

English speaker. I reply, "*You* are working. I am not. I am out to dinner in a restaurant." The immigrant worker is more likely to ask politely whether I am finished with my plate and whether I would like it removed.

If the work environment becomes calm enough to allow it, I value the opportunity to talk briefly with such immigrants. We can learn from them just as they learn from us. We can learn about the miseries they have fled, the hopes that animate them, the risks they have taken, the courage they have shown, the reverence they have for being where they can speak their minds or love whom they choose without fear of being murdered for doing so. We can also learn of the struggles they face here as they try to adjust to a new environment while remaining true to the parts of their own heritage that they value most. If we listen well, we are rewarded well by learning about ourselves—about what we do well and what we should strive to do better.

Sometimes I can show a bit of familiarity with an immigrant's homeland. I am often moved by how readily people respond and by the sense of loss they reveal, even if they have run for their lives. They miss sights and sounds, breezes and aromas, rhythms and rituals, songs and sunsets. They carry that with them, as gifts to us.

When we think about going out to dinner, or making something new and interesting at home, we ought to be mindful of how fortunate we are to have so many recent immigrants, including refugees, to enrich our gastronomic lives, our cultural awareness, and our understanding of ourselves. It's good food for thought.

6

GET IT IN WRITING

Statutory law, such as the Statute of Fraud, may require some kinds of contracts be put in writing and executed with particular formalities, for the contract to be enforceable. Otherwise, the parties may enter into a binding agreement without signing a formal written document. For example, Virginia Supreme Court has held in Lucy v. Zehmer that even an agreement made on a piece of napkin can be considered a valid contract, if the parties were both sane, and showed mutual assent and consideration.

—Cornell Law School Legal Information Institute (2023)

On April 13, 2021, Israeli police cut the speaker cables at the Al-Aqsa Mosque in Jerusalem, prompting protests, further police actions on May 7, and vindictive and devastating tribalist regression by both Jews and Arabs in the ancient town of Lod. That town saw many profound changes over the centuries, but in recent times its population of approximately 70,000 has been about 30 percent Arab, and despite structural inequality and discrimination, had mostly enjoyed neighborly civility and calm. Once its residents stopped seeing one another as members of the same moral community, all equally human despite their differences, explosive violence followed. Later, the ever combative and divisive Benjamin Netanyahu was ousted as Israeli Prime Minister by a coalition of radically differing constituencies. Now, after less than two years of roiling instability, he's back—at least for a while. Whether the residents of Lod can ever again embrace their common humanity and advance common interests is unknown; so far, the results are dismal, as Netanyahu has brought the country to the brink of civil war. Most of what lies ahead is unknowable.

My mother completed teacher training in 1929. Her younger sister, Bertha, became a social worker. Kamal Fahmy, scion of a prominent Egyptian family, came to graduate school at Harvard. I don't know how he and Bertha met; their marriage must have taken considerable explaining to her Jewish family and his Egyptian family. They settled in Cairo, where Bertha became Thoraya Fahmy and, to much acclaim, led the development of social work as a professional field in Egypt. For many years there was an explicit understanding that when I was old enough, I would visit them in Cairo. I looked forward eagerly to that adventure, perhaps after high school. But Kamal died in the crash of a private airplane in the 1950s. For more than 50 years I yearned to see Egypt. That dream remained deferred until a tour in 2011.

We started in Cairo, moved to the upper Nile, Luxor, the Valley of the Kings, and other important sites before heading back to Cairo and the pyramids. Suddenly, mysterious changes confused us all. News broadcasts that had been available ceased, our tour leaders seemed distressed and became less accessible, and we could not get answers about what was going on. It was the Arab Spring.

When we reached Cairo, our tour leader directed us not to leave the hotel or be on a balcony. We were to be packed and ready to leave at a moment's notice but might not have further instructions for days. All cell phone and internet connections were disabled. Through the windows we saw armed troops patrolling and smoke in the distance from burning cars. Tanks rumbled through the streets. All scheduled flights to and from the airport were canceled. Several days later an emergency evacuation got us out of Egypt, moments before the closure of the airport, to safety in Switzerland.

Earlier, that Egyptian tour leader had said this: "When I was young, my mother told me if I am doing business, I must always make a contract, get it in writing, all the details. Unless, she said, it is one of our Jewish neighbors. Then all you need is his word."

As I think about Lod, Cairo, and that guide's mother, I am more heartened than discouraged. These stories might warrant despair, yet they also reveal that ordinary people tend to get along peaceably until external forces of power or authority impose divisive influences on them. Treaties and cease-fire agreements are written reflections of deals that require more than anyone's word to create trust. Indeed, because such agreements are often violated, trust grows not when the agreements are announced but only as they are implemented. Absent effective enforcement, that might or might not happen. Contracts that enable business deals work in part because they are backed by functioning legal systems that make them enforceable. Getting it in writing, though not always sufficient, is typically a good idea.

When I was offered an appointment in 1972 as philosophy chair at the University of Maryland, College Park, and charged to build a strong and distinctive department, I was promised many things. These included a plan to hire ten additional professors. I asked that the plan be endorsed in writing. The appointing officer said that was unnecessary. "My word is good," he affirmed. I replied, "If a man's word is good, it ought to be equally good on paper. I do want it in writing." When I arrived in the fall, he was gone. His successor had misgivings about the plans, and especially the large number of new faculty appointments. He proposed negotiating about some of the items. I brandished a copy of the letter, said there was nothing to negotiate as these were settled matters, and that we should make five appointments in the first year. With support from faculty in the department, I required that faculty applicants have a master's degree or equivalent in a field outside philosophy, in keeping with my focus on philosophy's relevance to other fields. Of those five appointments, two were African American, two were women, one was Asian-American; one held a master's in physics and another a master's in biology. These many varieties of diversity secured the administration's resolve to continue strong support for the department's development. Having the plans in writing was essential.

When asked to join Syracuse University in 1986 as dean of arts and sciences, I thought, wrongly, that I knew what I needed to know about such negotiations. I obtained written commitments of all sorts, including substantial funds for grants to improve the quality of faculty life within their departments. The person who appointed me, the previous arts and sciences dean, had moved on as vice-chancellor. When I arrived, I found that he had taken everything with him to his new position. I mean *everything*. He took the two associate deans, his secretary, all the furniture. My office was a totally empty room; there was not even a telephone. I had to find a different office to make a call to begin my Campaign of

Complaint. I ought to have been far more careful and complete about what I got in writing. But I'm not certain it would have sufficed, on a napkin or otherwise.

The offices were not all I found empty. The chemistry and physics departments were all male; geology had one woman (who remained its only woman for sixteen years). Biology had some women, mostly teaching botany and other subjects that the chemists and physicists disdained as not real science anyway. In resolving to change all this, I faced an intransigent chemistry department and a vice-chancellor, himself a former chemist, who questioned the need for a biology department that was more than a small service unit. But he listened as I argued for investing in the life sciences, and we then developed an ambitious and detailed plan. I knew that to use that plan effectively in recruiting, I needed it in writing. It was signed by the chancellor, the vice-chancellor, and me as dean. On the basis of that excellent plan, we made four superb initial appointments, including senior biologists who resigned from tenured positions and moved to Syracuse. Then, in an abrupt reversal, the vice-chancellor informed me that we would abandon the plan, directing me to tell the biology department chair. I did so; his incendiary rage was fully justified and long enduring. Getting commitments in writing can be crucial but cannot prevent subsequent betrayals of trust.

Even asking for written commitments can connote a lack of trust and undermine further trust. Within a family, co-workers, or a circle of friends, such a request can be deeply offending. Sometimes getting it in writing is essential, sometimes it's just a good idea, sometimes it's completely inappropriate. Making that judgment often involves uncertainty and some risk. I'm not aware of any algorithms or rules that can eliminate that risk. If I hear of any, I'll want to get them in writing.

7

FOURTH GRADE MATH, A SUPER BOWL RING, AND TOO MANY OFFICES

"I'm late! I'm late! For a very important date! No time to say 'hello,' 'goodbye!' I'm late! I'm late! I'm late!"

—*The White Rabbit*, lyrics by Bob Hilliard, 1951

It seemed unjust when, in the fourth grade, I was banned from the daily mathematics exercise. There's a reason to tell you about this, but that will take some doing. It's not for self-aggrandizement; quite the contrary. The exercise was this: the teacher voiced a long, rapid-fire problem, such as "6 plus 3 divided by 3 times 9 plus 3 is equal to what?" Whoever first raised a hand was called on. This seemed pretty thin stuff to me, and I always shot my hand up as soon as the teacher got to "is." I then would give the right answer, prompting an "Oh, not again" groan from classmates. The teacher put a stop to it by banning me from the game. I wanted to cry "foul," but she made the rules.

I've always been a quick responder, impatient when the driver in front takes a long time to react to a green light, and fast off the blocks as a high school sprinter. That was for a 50-yard dash. I couldn't even finish a 100-yard dash. I had academic tenacity, but physically it was fast reflexes and little stamina.

Days after I joined Syracuse University as dean of arts and sciences in August 1986, I went to an annual retreat for high-level administrators at the university's magnificent Minnowbrook Conference Center on Blue Mountain Lake in the Adirondack Mountains. We had meetings of various kinds and abundant recreation—including a traditional volleyball game. I joined that game, as did George Burman, the incoming Management School dean whom I had not yet met. I was in the third row, defending, as the opposing server drove the ball toward us. Immediately, there followed a puzzling and disconcerting visual experience. In a fraction of a second, I saw a static image—everyone in place awaiting the serve—except for one large guy in the front row streaking across that static scene toward where the ball was heading. It was like watching special effects in a movie. A second later the scene unfroze, and everyone was in motion. But that initial reactor was already in place, awaiting the ball to spike it back over the net. I couldn't make sense of what I had seen.

Later I learned that the exceptional athleticism I had witnessed was George Burman in action, long after a career in the National Football League earned him a Super Bowl Ring. He still had uncanny reflexes that showed the rest of us what swift reactions are like at the highest levels of human performance. With a Ph.D. in economics from the University of Chicago, he was now the third NFL player I had met and the second (after Frank Ryan) who was also an academic star. I no longer thought of myself as having fast reactions.

Part of what had been so impressive in George's move was its astonishing swiftness. A second part was that he went to exactly the right spot. He did not figure that out as he analyzed the situation; he just did it, using that portion of the brain that Daniel Kahneman, in *Thinking, Fast and Slow*, describes as functioning independently of any reflection or analysis. Also, he demonstrated exquisitely sharp powers of detection. We all react to what we sense in various ways, but some detectors are sharper than others. An MRI yields a sharper image than an x-ray; a CT-scan is a still sharper detector. Before George's reflexes could propel him into motion, he had to perceive the serve accurately. The sharpness of his visual detection made that possible. A throughgoing objective in the courses I teach and co-teach is to induce students to sharpen their detectors—all of them—as much as possible, to enable them more effectively to pursue whatever goals they have.

In a batting cage, my octogenarian reflexes (as of August 2022) enable me to contact most pitches at 35 miles per hour. At 45 mph I miss most. At 50 I rarely even see them: the first detection is the thump of the pitch hitting the screen behind me. Major League hitters must react in a small fraction of a second and frequently hit pitches at speeds in excess of 90 or even 100 mph. They don't decide whether or not to swing. They just swing, or they don't. Burman-like, they combine superbly sharp detectors and astonishing athletic skill with internalized judgment about how to use that skill effectively. After the game, they may study videos of their times at bat, analyze bat plane angles, consider whether a slightly different bat weight should be tried, and consult with others, using various cognitive strategies that typify thinking slow by drawing on other parts of their brains. Every situation in which we can act one way or another has these components, but when the need to act is not time-sensitive, we often overlook the powerful influence our swift initial impressions have on our later reflective thinking.

These athletic stories are broadly useful metaphors. We had a math major on the ice hockey team. That's a rare mix. He emphasized that many teammates were stronger on the ice, faster and tougher. Yet he was highly successful. His specialty in mathematics was pattern recognition, and he used his insights from that field to perceive what patterns were emerging on the ice and to anticipate where he should be, rather than just reacting to where the puck was, instant by instant. In doing that so well, he was crucial to the team's success. In almost any domain, people with the ability to perceive emerging patterns have an advantage over those who are simply reacting to instantaneous perceptions.

George and I became good friends. Our differences in backgrounds and politics were of no consequence because we were university allies. I learned much from him about injuries, recovery, and long-term damage to athletes. He may have learned some things from me about liberal education and academic strategies.

After being dean, I taught some courses in Public Administration, spent three years teaching half-time at the SUNY Upstate Medical University, and then accepted a one-year appointment at Yale as visiting professor of philosophy and bioethicist in residence. In May 2004, my situation changed radically. Debbie Freund—a distinguished and quick-thinking "get it done" scholar of health policy—arrived as a new vice chancellor for academic affairs and the university's first provost. She swiftly replaced the arts and sciences dean with Cathryn Newton. At their request, I met with them in Debbie's office, where they urged me to lead a thorough reformation of a sadly foundering old honors program. I declined, explaining that I would not even be in Syracuse. I had an apartment in New Haven, fall classes scheduled and enrolled, and only a few weeks to clear out my medical school office, move to New Haven, and begin my year there. They accepted my reasoning.

About ten days later they asked to see me again; I presumed that was to seek my advice about who might best do that honors program job, and perhaps whom to avoid. I was pleased by that prospect. To my dismay, they said, "We understand about this Yale thing. But you have to do the honors program. There's no acceptable alternative." My protests were futile. Within days I was named founding director of the Renée Crown University Honors Program, charged to create a nationally important and exemplary program.

What has that to do with George, you well may wonder.

I had a philosophy department office, my medical school office, my new honors program office, the home office in which I did all my writing, and my office at Yale. As I was walking by the Management School, George emerged and asked how I was doing. I said, "George, I'm struggling. I now have five offices and I have no idea where anything is." George rose to his full NFL height, looked way down at me with an aura of pride and smug superiority, and said, "I accomplish *that* with just one office."

I divided my time between the two full-time jobs at Syracuse and Yale. People who knew of this lunatic schedule often asked what I listened to during the weekly four-and-a-half-hour drive each way. They wondered about books on tape (actual tapes in those pre-digital days), music, news broadcasts, and more. My response was unexpected. I acknowledged listening to NPR, the BBC, some music, and a few other things. But mostly I turned that all off and cherished the silence. Constant auditory input exacts a price; it can distract us from our own thoughts. Silence, and respect for silence, can pay great dividends. The film *Nomadland* has a brilliant soundtrack in part because the director was unafraid to let visual images speak for themselves at times, in silence. The classic museum robbery film *Topkapi* also employs silence to increase the dramatic tension. And there's a superbly effective use of silence in *CODA*, allowing the viewers to understand somewhat more fully the experience of deaf people. I sometimes tell students (forbidden to have earphones or other listening devices) to do absolutely nothing until I signal otherwise, and then I remain silent for 90 seconds. They grow increasingly uncomfortable. When they estimate how long the silent interval was, they tend to overestimate it significantly. I ask them to volunteer their thoughts; many report recognizing anxieties, having creative ideas, or puzzling about a question new to them.

On my drives, I used silence to plan classes, let my mind wander, imagine humiliating retribution against tailgaters, notice the way the fading light filters through the trees, see creatures in the clouds and imagine seeing them as the pre-scientific ancients did. Silence nourishes serendipity. Sometimes I realized with surprise that I was thinking about a new idea that later appeared as an op-ed. Often, at each stop, I would capture these thoughts by making notes before driving off. Those silent intervals were among the most gratifying and productive times every week. (Among my eccentricities is aversion to noise; I won't patronize loud restaurants and don't like background music when I work. People differ in that respect.)

I've long opposed the common practice among busy administrators of scheduling back-to-back meetings all day, arguing instead for built-in breaks—for themselves and their support staff—to provide restorative moments and perhaps even a few interludes of silence to foster actual thought. When primatologist Jane Goodall visited, I was dismayed by her schedule. I said, "Jane, it's 7 p.m. and you've been running non-stop since 6:30 this morning, first at the lakeshore with indigenous colleagues, then visiting local schools, giving presentations in classes, meeting with researchers. It's too much. Why not have your schedulers put several breaks into your program each day?" She brightened, and with wide-eyed surprise, replied, "Oh! Then I could go to the loo!"

Conversations, like volleyball, involve passing something back and forth by turns. When a receiver anticipates what's coming and reacts, the result can interrupt a speaker who would have preferred silent, attentive listening. It's well known that in clinical situations, male physicians interrupt patients more frequently than women physicians do, but don't get as much useful information from those more aggressive inquiries. Active, attentive listening is hard work, requiring patience, focus, and energy. Also, the impulsive reaction is often wrong: the ball isn't headed where you thought it was. Speech is linear—one word follows another—whereas we think many thoughts simultaneously in parallel, with a kind of split-screen imagery. Thus, as I started writing these pages, I had many possible threads in mind and even as I wrote I wondered how they might best be woven into something linear on the page. Would they seem to be careening around like a puck on ice, or would patterns emerge that made sense?

Similarly, when I listen carefully to a speaker, I typically imagine, as I hear the start of a sentence, many possibilities for how that sentence might end. I wait with curiosity to see whether any of those is forthcoming. *Being* silent, as well as *having* silence, can pay important dividends. It can facilitate listening and also signal that one is listening. Once, as dean, I talked with a frustrated administrator (at a level above mine) about the general perception of that person as not a good listener. "I'm a *very* good listener!" was affirmed in defiant defense. I replied:

> First, maybe you are a good listener when you're listening. But when you are in transmitter mode, rather than receiver mode, people have no idea when that will end or how to flip that

switch, short of swinging a two-by-four at you. So there's an initial impression that you're not interested in listening. But let's stipulate that you are listening, with complete comprehension and reliable recall. Second, you're often multi-tasking, glancing at your cell phone, flipping pages, avoiding eye-contact. So even if we stipulate . . . however well you are listening, the impression you give is that you're not listening. Third, even if you are as good as you claim at listening, you need to learn how to convey a credible impression of really paying attention to the speaker. Without that, you'll keep your reputation as a poor listener.

Whether those comments had any lasting effect remains unclear. At least they gained concurrence in principle and a promise to try to put them into practice. Changing behavioral characteristics like that, however, takes much more than good will. Just as the athlete, musician, surgeon, or any other professional must spend long hours repeating desirable actions until they become finely honed and habitual, sustained mindful practice is also essential for improved listening skills.

That fourth-grade math class was not just about arithmetic. Any slight lapse of focus would have made getting the right answer impossible. So it was also about attentive listening—early training in sharpening our detectors. Few people can earn Super Bowl rings, no matter how hard they try. Everyone can learn the uses and benefits of silence, can work to be an ever-better listener, and can strive to keep sharpening all their detectors. Now, so many decades later, I suspect that my fourth-grade math teacher knew it and was doing what she could to nudge us in that direction.

8

MISSILES, NOTES,
AND A JOLLY PINK GIANT

---

*"Once the rockets are up, Who cares where they come
down? That's not my department," says Wernher von Braun.*

From "Wernher von Braun," by Tom Lehrer
(*That Was the Year that Was*, 1965)

Nina Byers, the pioneering particle physicist who became a leading force for opening physics to women, was at Stanford when
I arrived as a new graduate student in 1960. (The next year she left
for UCLA where she spent the rest of her luminous career.) She
had posted a notice seeking a grader for her quantum mechanics course; I applied. She'd expected physics students, not a student in philosophy. But I had studied quantum mechanics at
MIT with Victor Weisskopf (who invoked Plato in teaching
physics, and later received the Presidential Medal of Science),
and that was enough to get an interview. I was sure that other
applicants were better qualified, just not better credentialed.

The interview reinforced my sense of being an imposter. She gave me a problem and asked how I would grade answers to it. I stared at it in bewilderment, then nervously said, "I don't see this as a quantum mechanics problem at all. It's dressed up in the language of quantum mechanics. But all I can see is classical mechanics; a billiard ball problem." To my amazement and terror, she said, "Right. You're hired." Suddenly, I was a physics grader. My MIT classmate Alan Ardell, doing his doctorate at Stanford in materials science, helped me muddle through the grading. I'm still grateful. Byers left the following year for UCLA. Alan, after a brief stint at Caltech, also went to UCLA; he's now Professor Emeritus there. Byers had been a Fellow of Somerville College at Oxford, a progressive college for women that produced many distinguished scholars who were important and effective opponents of academic misogyny. Philippa Foot, whom you will meet in Chapter 21, is among them.

In the spring following the grading venture, I applied for a summer job at Lockheed Aircraft in nearby Sunnyvale. Once again, MIT credentials paved the way. I was appointed as associate engineer, in the Midas Satellite program within the Missiles and Space Division, starting on June 8, 1961. But this time I may have been overqualified. Mostly, I worked as a technical writer and was asked to produce the annual report for our section. When I submitted it, days before the due date, my supervisor complained that it was shorter than parallel reports by his peers in other sections. He asked me to expand it. I asked whether any substantive point, large or small, was omitted. There was not; he just wanted a longer report. I said I would not make the writing worse by padding it with flab, but he could do so as he saw fit.

A few days later, I saw a way to strengthen one point in that report but was denied access to it on the grounds that my security clearance was not sufficient to allow me to see it. It had been reclassified at a higher level. I pointed out that as its author, I knew exactly what was in it, so there could be no security risk in my seeing it. My argument failed—a Wiener's Warning moment (that will be explained in the next chapter). The work environment became unpleasant as I turned to other tasks, with new understanding of how private contractors and the U.S. Air Force Air Defense Command Program, at least sometimes, wobbled along together. I was "laid off" on July 28, 1961. I can't tell you about what was in that report, because even now that would violate my obligations under federal law.

In 1964, as a new assistant professor at Western Reserve University (about to join with Case Institute of Technology, as detailed in Chapter 16), I was prompted to recall those episodes from graduate school. My office was in a building that was physically austere, but rich in characters. Among them was Ray Nelson, an immense, ruddy man proud of his Swedish heritage, whose talents radiated in all directions. He was a professor in philosophy and in mathematics, and he was also a computer scientist. He was a superb, self-taught jazz pianist who learned by playing 78 rpm records over and over and trying to play what he heard. He was an irrepressible font of wisdom and good humor. We called him the Jolly Pink Giant.

He would walk into my office without a knock or a word, stride to the blackboard, write something, and silently leave. One day it was, "Make lists, then your life will be better, like mine." (I've been making lists—on 3 x 5 cards—ever since.) Another day it was, "When you are dealing with a dummy, watch out." As a physics grader, I was the dummy and was lucky to escape unscathed. At Lockheed, I was dealing with a dummy and should have watched out more carefully.

Also on our floor was a young mathematician who later did important work in several branches of pure and applied mathematics. He was Frank Ryan, who taught only morning classes because in the afternoons he was the quarterback of the Cleveland Browns—with whom he had a long and distinguished career. He was the first professional football player I had met (long before I met George Burman).

Ryan and Nelson were vivid exemplars of generalized excellence, of the possibility of many different talents finding expression in the life of a single person. Another Nelson also would emerge as an unexpected part of my story. Ray's daughter Susan Nelson (now Susan McGuire) was one of those youngsters whose every movement was a dance step, and she danced her way right to the top. She was a principal with the Martha Graham Dance Company, then with the Paul Taylor Dance Company, and then she became leader of the Taylor 2 Company. Seeing her dance with the Taylor company in Washington, D.C. ignited my interest in modern dance. Later she brought the Taylor 2 Company to Syracuse University—an inspiring experience for our thousands of students interested in dance. On April 15, 2006, the Paul Taylor Company was in Syracuse for the world premiere of *Troilus and Cressida (Reduced)*, a work commissioned by then Dean Cathryn Newton. Paul was familiar with and enthusiastic about her work on the science of shipwrecks. As I talked with him during that visit about our common interest in such maritime matters, I was reminded again of the powerful influence of the unpredictable connections among people and among ideas that can take us unawares and set us on unanticipated adventures of discovery and accomplishment. Susan McGuire, too, has been reflecting about those unplanned transitions as she nears completion of a book she is writing about her life in dance. Taylor's works were choreographed with meticulous detail; every movement of every part of each dancer's body was a product of his artistic genius and demanding craftsmanship combined with the talent and dedication of the dancers. It's not like that as we "dance" through life. However hard we may try to choreograph our own futures, we all have to rely on unexpected improvisation over and over again.

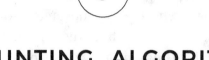

ACCOUNTING, ALGORITHMS, AND AGONIES

The significance of Smoot's ear is that it is a built-in error; it recognizes that fallibility is ever present in human affairs.

—Robert Tavernor (2007)

Norbert Wiener—creator of cybernetics, a field he described as "control and communication in the animal and the machine,"—left a wake of legends wherever he went. In one, he was walking along the vast multi-building passage at MIT called "The Infinite Corridor." Halfway, under the iconic Great Dome, he was greeted enthusiastically by a visiting former student walking the opposite way. They discussed mathematics until the former student was out of time. Wiener then said, "Do you recall, when we met just now, which way I was walking?" The visitor pointed. Wiener replied, "Oh, good! Then I've had my lunch."

Wiener's office was in the same building as my advisor's. One day Wiener and I entered the elevator at the basement level. It stopped at one; he started out. I said it was not yet his floor. He backed in. The same at two. At three, I said "This is your floor, sir." He said, "Thank you," left, and possibly headed toward his office. That one encounter lent credence to all the legends I had heard.

Wiener was both absent-minded and brilliant. He had a swift start, enrolling at Tufts University at eleven. A college graduate at fourteen, he studied zoology at Harvard and philosophy at Cornell before returning to Harvard as a doctoral student in mathematics, receiving his Ph.D. at nineteen. He was a font of wisdom. In a public lecture, I heard him urge caution against becoming controlled by information systems we invent to support our efforts. I call this *Wiener's Warning*. Grading students is one such system. When we grade, we use a system invented for that purpose. The simplest is *Pass/Fail*; the most complex is probably a scale from 0 to 100. Any choice about how to grade will disadvantage some students and benefit others. Those who excel may prefer fine distinctions and those who struggle may favor rough categories. Proposals to change a grading system always unleash howls of protest. Long ago, universities used letters, A to F, with + and - as refinements. Grade reports were handwritten. Then a more efficient, computerized system was adopted, which printed grade reports automatically. A student with a mathematics course grade of 99 asked his professor how that could be, when the student had 100 percent on every graded work all term. The professor inquired and was told by the Registrar that the system only generates two digits. "I've never had a student who did perfect work all semester," the professor replied. "But this student earned 100, and I insist that he get 100. I won't be ruled by that new system." The tenacious professor prevailed; the Registrar issued a handwritten grade report for that single student. It was just one small point, but it illustrates Wiener's large cautionary point lucidly.

Wiener's Warning served me well in my third year of graduate school. I was offered a dissertation fellowship that would cover my tuition, pay a stipend, and allow me to work full time on my dissertation. I declined it in favor of a teaching assistantship with the same stipend that required me to teach half time. I loved teaching, always learned from it, and knew I would write more effectively if I had something else to do when writing stalled. At the end of that third year, after I had successfully defended my dissertation and completed all the other academic requirements, I was puzzled to receive a bill for a half year of tuition. When I claimed this must be an error, the dean of graduate studies, a distinguished statistician who certainly knew how to count things, explained that the doctorate required three years of residency, but I had only two and a half years. Residency, he revealed, was calculated on the basis of tuition paid. Incredulous, I replied, "Are you saying that if I had accepted the dissertation fellowship to work full time on writing, I would not owe anything, but because I taught for you half time while writing my dissertation you now expect me to pay this large bill?" He confirmed this: that's how the accounting system worked, there was nothing more he could do.

With Wiener as my muse, I replied that I would never pay that bill, but would go forth without the doctorate and tell the story of this duplicitous absurdity as often and as widely as I could. I added that if the bill had to be paid, he should find the funds himself. Sadly, he responded, he had no access to any funds that could be used that way. I stormed out of his office muttering something about extortion, not expecting to hear from him again. But several days later he contacted me to propose that we negotiate a settlement. He would cover half the bill if I agreed to pay the other half. I quietly pointed out that by his own account, he had access to no funds that could be used that way. Either this new offer was a scam, or he had not told the truth earlier. That ended the conversation. Somehow, consulting with the Philosophy Department, he resolved the problem and I received my doctorate in 1963. That was his last year as dean of graduate studies. The following year he was chancellor of the City University of New York (CUNY), the first of several major university leadership positions to come.

About a decade later, when I chaired the Philosophy Department at the University of Maryland, College Park, Wiener's Warning again paid off. Under legislative pressure, the University imposed a faculty reporting requirement. We were told to complete daily activity reports, indicating for every hour whether it was an hour of teaching (T), service (S), or research (R). I had been asked by then Congressman Albert Gore, Jr. to testify before the House Committee on Science and Technology's Subcommittee on Investigations and Oversight. That required presenting an initial statement followed by responses to questions. I drafted my statement and used it for discussion in a graduate seminar. The students critiqued the draft and envisioned questions I might be asked. After the hearings, I revised that statement for publication; it appeared in a professional journal. I described this activity, returning the blank reporting form to the administration— adding that I would complete it only after they determined whether that time in class was T, S, or R, with an explanation of how they decided. I never heard from them again and did no activity reports. No harm came to me or my department colleagues as a result.

Evaluating a professor's case for tenure raises some of the same thorny issues as grading students. Candidates are assessed for their teaching, research, and service potential, with their contributions to date providing most of the evidence. Predictions of future performance are notoriously unreliable, however, and those who evaluate candidates typically disagree about how such predictions should be made. An unusually powerful and persuasive account of these difficulties—in all fields—appears in *Noise: A Flaw in Human Judgment* (Daniel Kahneman, Oliver Sibony, and Cass R. Sunstein, 2021). These authors distinguish between rules, such as "Do not drive faster than 65 miles per hour," and standards, such as "Do not drive recklessly or at speeds inappropriate to the circumstances." Rules provide clarity, requiring only an assessment of the facts. Standards require judgment, inviting conflict and inconsistency. It's easy to determine how many books or articles a professor has published. It is harder to assess the quality of the journals, the significance of the work, and the future stability or importance of the professor's interests. Kahneman et al. favor rules and algorithms, arguing that if they are inadequate for the decisions at issue, the solution is not to give up but to develop better algorithms—although they also are clear about the costs and limitations of using or improving algorithms.

Assume that research has confirmed that students who sing in a residence hall shower take longer to emerge, causing other students to wait longer for access to the shower. The students adopt a rule banning singing in the shower. Boomer Loudlung then spends thirty minutes in the shower, humming his favorite arias. Brought before the Disciplinary Council, he pleads "not guilty," claiming he was not singing, just humming. How would the Council members react?

One might claim he's guilty because he was producing vocal music in a manner obviously chosen to circumvent the legislative intent or because humming should be understood as a species of singing. A defender might hold that singing allows for producing recognizable phonemes of speech, which humming does not, so he can't possibly have violated the ban on singing by humming. The advocate of standards might propose the following: "Let's use our discretion. He was trying to get away with something and we shouldn't allow that. He's guilty." Another member might say, "We have to acquit him, but then must revise the rule so it explicitly includes humming as a violation." This debate about how to think about the case has costs in time, energy, and possibly good will. With no resolution when the meeting time ran out, another Disciplinary Council session was scheduled for the following week. Each member was charged to reflect independently on all aspects of the case, taking care not to communicate with one another about it nor to reach any overall judgment about the outcome. Loudlung went back to his room to practice whistling.

I made up the case about humming; I did not make up the Covid pandemic. As a member of the New York State Task Force on Life and the Law, I had participated in 2015 in the development of guidelines for the allocation of ventilators in the case of a possible pandemic. Following a 2019 article in *The New Yorker* that cited my role on the Task Force, I heard from high school and college classmates I had not heard from in many decades and was approached by news media from Australia to Europe. In the Task Force meetings, I had been a strong advocate of developing and disclosing clear guidelines for the use of ventilators. In 2019, I was repeatedly asked what rules I favored for making these tragic choices—choices where every possible option is bad. I replied that ventilators must not be thought of in isolation, but as part of an ecosystem including trained staff and necessary materials. If any of that array is missing, the ventilators are to no avail. More importantly, I emphasized that our tragic choices cannot be dispelled or fully resolved by any decisional algorithm.

One reporter invoked the economist's beloved metric of Quality Adjusted Life Years (QALY), seeking agreement about this hypothetical: *Consider an octogenarian with Covid-19 and various co-morbidities on a ventilator, with uncertain outcome. An otherwise healthy 40-year-old also needed a ventilator, but none was free.* The reporter thought it clear that to maximize benefit to public health, the right decision—tragic to be sure—would be to move the elderly person to the best palliative care, knowing that this person would almost certainly die as a result, and give the younger person the ventilator. This would be required by QALY guidelines that make probability of recovery determinative. The reporter was audibly startled by my response.

If the elderly person is Ruth Bader Ginsburg, I replied, there's a credible case that maximizing public health requires doing everything possible to keep her alive, even for just a year. I did not insist on this choice—only that a credible case could be made for it. No algorithm, guidelines, or rules could determine the merits of that case. That would require a judgment in which one's values and experience, as well as the empirical evidence, would mix and matter. This is so in every tragic-choice situation; there is always an ineliminable need at some point for judgment that no algorithm can replace. (A second example could be Oprah Winfrey, also much beloved, whose contributions to social justice and the public good are beyond measure.)

I conveyed my views to Kahneman, quoting the exchange with the reporter, and referencing a recent excerpt from *Noise* in the *Harvard Business Review*:

However . . . I have some misgivings about the claim that algorithms are always at least as good as judgment. Recently, after a barrage of inquiries from the press, I wrote a piece about ventilator allocation guidelines that addressed related issues. I'd be curious about your reactions to this excerpt. (I agree that reducing misery is a far better goal for policy than maximizing "happiness" . . . whatever that is, and that deferring intuition heightens its utility.)

He replied as expected:

Sam,

As you probably guessed, I don't agree with you. Algorithms and people make different mistakes; people make more of them. The mistakes that algorithms make strike us as absurd, and we rarely get the algorithm's opinion of the human mistakes. We know from existing evidence that the expected value of the outcomes is worse when people can override the algorithm than if the algorithm is given the last words. How many people would die by human mistakes to avoid the extraordinarily unlikely outcome of taking RBG off a ventilator? A better solution than using judgment at the end of the process is to improve the coding system, perhaps using judgment to describe some cases as exceptionally important. Or at least that's my two cents about the problem.

Of course, we must recognize that algorithms are often abhorrent and will not be used even if they do a better job than humans. It is hard for people to admit that the faculty of which they are most proud—the ability to integrate complex information—is where they are most noisy and error-prone.

Best, Danny

Tenure committee discussions can have some of the same features and should adopt "Noise hygiene" measures as Kahneman et al. advise. These include agreeing on what factors are relevant, considering each such factor independently, limiting discussion to those factors, discussing each case multiple times, and deferring any overall judgment about a case until the end. And yet . . . there's no protection against the last minute surprise, such as new information: that the candidate has engaged in unacceptable behavior (was it culpable harassment or a distressing but atypical indiscretion—should it derail the case?); that a staff member reporting to the candidate was using university resources to support a small private business (not with the candidate's approval but with the candidate's knowledge); that aspects of the candidate's publication record were discovered to overstate the case (carelessness by a busy researcher or culpable fraud?). These are real examples.

In some ways, these academic decisions are of a recurrent kind; yet each is singular in being about a unique candidate. Medical decisions have this duality also; each case is one example of a general kind, yet each patient is a unique individual for whom typical reactions may not be appropriate. A striking difference between the two categories, however, is that personnel decisions can be made according to a timetable determined by the organization. Clinical choices require decisions according to a timetable determined by the clinical realities, sometimes within hours or even minutes, drawing on the experience and training of those with the burden of decision.

Granting the central thesis of *Noise*—that, overall, algorithms and rules are more reliable than human judgment—there remain domains and situations in which it's hard to imagine any approach other than judgment. One can agree that there are better and worse ways to prepare for judgment, that the processes of judgment can be sloppy or rigorous, and that some people are better equipped than others—by qualities of mind and discernment—to make successful judgments reliably. But in the end, there's no avoiding it.

I have a talented young friend who evaluates proposals for a major animation studio. She doesn't consider uninvited pitches; initial screening brings her only proposals already assessed as having good potential. She can then send them into a complex process that may lead to production, or she can turn them down. No proposal advances without her approval. I can't imagine how that could be automated.

The same applies to casting directors. The success or failure of a show depends crucially on who fills the roles. Casting is a creative art that draws on deep knowledge, interpersonal insight, and negotiating skills. When it's done at its best, viewers don't see the actors; they only see, and believe in, the characters. Guidelines can help set the goals and avoid disaster, but the final choice is no job for an algorithm.

And then there's book publishing. Among my treasures is a batch of letters from more than a dozen publishers turning down my proposal in the early 1970s for a medical ethics textbook. No such text existed then. The letters have a discouraging consistency: "This is an intriguing idea but we're sorry, we've looked into the possibilities and there's no viable market for this. There's no field called 'medical ethics' or 'bioethics' and no courses in college or university catalogs listed that way, so nobody we can sell this book to." Finally, one publisher decided, with clear anxiety, to take the risk. By the following year, *Moral Problems in Medicine* was adopted at more than a hundred colleges and universities. My reaction was that publishers haven't a clue about how to deal with something unfamiliar to them. They could be trained to do better, but not replaced by automation.

That guidelines are sometimes insufficient doesn't mean they are useless or even not essential. However, the moment when one faces a tragic choice is too late to begin thinking about how to decide. We should pursue better guidelines and also improve the training of those who might have to exercise judgment in time-sensitive situations. When our guidelines are inconclusive or lead to decisions that violate or undermine our values, we can hear and heed Norbert Wiener's voice because we carry that with us. We can chuckle at his eccentricities and marvel at his mathematical genius, but we need always venerate the wisdom and insight of Wiener's Warning.

TWO PIPES, TWO CIGARETTES, AND ONE CIGAR

A custom loathsome to the eye, hateful to the nose, harmful to the brain, dangerous to the lungs, and in the black stinking fume thereof, nearest resembling the horrible Stigian smoke of the pit that is bottomless.

—King James 1, *A Counterblast to Tobacco*, 1604

Niels Bohr sat at the front of our classroom facing the students, in a chair with a writing tablet on its left side. In the first row, I had an unobstructed view of the Danish Nobel Laureate physicist who, to MIT students, ranked only with Einstein as deities beyond compare. This gentle septuagenarian held a pipe in his left hand; on the tablet was a large box of wooden matches. In 1920 Bohr had said, "When it comes to atoms, language can be used only as in poetry. The poet, too, is not nearly so concerned with describing facts as with creating images." Contemporary art had left the representational styles of the past behind and was creating images that puzzled and provoked the viewer. So I asked Bohr if he had any reaction to current trends in the visual arts.

I dimly recall that he started to speak of complementarity between the work and the viewer as the experience such art is meant to induce. But I quickly lost concentration on what he was saying. His pipe had burned out. He had taken a wooden match from the box, struck it deftly, and held it steady in his right hand. He did not light the pipe. He was totally absorbed in thought. As he spoke, the flame burned along the match toward his hand. I watched with dismay until that flame was so close that he felt the heat, shook the match vigorously to extinguish the flame, and tossed the spent match to the floor. Without pause in his comments, he repeated the process, igniting another match and again holding it without remembering to light the pipe, and again rescuing his hand by dropping the spent match. By then I was completely, hypnotically focused on the minuet of matches. I have not forgotten what Bohr said—I did not even hear it.

Back then, faculty could smoke as they saw fit in classes. A few years later, in graduate school, I was a teaching assistant for Donald Davidson—a complex polymath who excelled in the performing arts, aviation, athletics, scholarship, and teaching. As a student at Harvard, he had played duets with Leonard Bernstein, who wrote the score for Davidson's production of Aristophanes' *The Birds*. Davidson did not typically smoke in class. However, one day in an epistemology course, discussing Hume's views about causation, he lit a filtered cigarette and from time to time paused to take a leisurely puff and blow the smoke toward the ceiling. An ash tray sat unused on the table in front of him. With each puff, the ash grew longer but did not fall. The longer it grew, the harder it was to attend to anything else. By the time the ash was more than half the length of the cigarette, few students were hearing a word. I scanned their faces; they all seemed to be staring at the cigarette with rapt, bewildered focus, much as I had been transfixed when watching Bohr. When the ash reached the filter, Davidson held the cigarette aloft and said, approximately:

> Hume knew that our causal judgments rely on the assumption that the future will conform to the past. He also knew that assumption might be false—that what we expect, based on our experience, may not be what happens.

And Davidson and his cigarette, ash intact, left the room.

Preparing for that class, he had straightened a paper clip into a small, straight rod and inserted it into the cigarette, creating an armature to hold the ash in place. His background in theater created an unforgettable moment for that class and reinforced my conviction that teaching is a performing art. Getting a point right is pointless if one fails to get that point across.

That's one pipe and one cigarette. I didn't have much to do with cigars, nor did I appreciate how important they could be even to people who were not Winston Churchill, George Burns, or Fidel Castro. When I arrived at Syracuse as Arts and Sciences Dean, I attended the conference at Minnowbrook, described in Chapter 7. I asked Chancellor Eggers to bar smoking in the meetings. He said that most participants were not smokers, that only a few were. I replied, "Then, Sir, I'm sorry to say that you will be meeting without your new Dean of Arts and Sciences." So he announced that as a courtesy to some participants, the meetings would be smoke-free; this angered a few old-timers, but they did not challenge Eggers.

The deans of the various schools and colleges met monthly for dinner and conversation. I was invited to join that group and eagerly accepted, noting that I assumed there would not be smoking at these events. I had come from the Washington, D.C. area where there was no need for such a question but learned at Minnowbrook that my new colleagues had no such constraints. Although the group readily acceded to my request, Richard Oliker, Dean of the Management School, said he'd be damned if he'd go to a dinner where he couldn't smoke his cigar, and he dropped out of the group. That's the cigar.

The Newhouse School of Public Communication has long had close collaborative relations with Arts and Sciences. Their dean, Ed Stevens, invited me to meet with them shortly after my arrival. I'd been writing op-eds for the *Los Angeles Times* and *The Washington Post* and doing some work on films for PBS, so I viewed that faculty as kindred spirits. One of them was John Keats, whose work I had read and admired. Ed introduced me to his faculty, requesting a smoke-free meeting. Keats rose, lit a cigarette, sauntered to the front of the room, blew some smoke, and said, "Well, I'd rather go out and smoke than stay in here and listen to *this* guy." And out he strode. He did have a way with words.

The second pipe was in the hand of my colleague Ed Gettier at Wayne State University during my first year after graduate school. Ed smoked it constantly and seemed busily occupied with the related paraphernalia:—a tamping tool, pipe cleaners, a tobacco pouch. No wooden matches for him. He used what seemed like a miniature flame thrower, a small torch that hissed and projected a focused flame into the bowl of the pipe, quickly igniting the tobacco. Our offices, in an

old house, had little acoustical privacy. Hearing an agonizing howl, I bolted into Ed's office. He had meant to relight his
pipe, but the bowl was empty; he'd smoked all the tobacco.
When he aimed the flame and puffed the pipe, he inhaled
that flame and blistered his throat. The future had not con-
formed to the past. I'm not sure he ever smoked again.

Tobacco has played an important role in commerce,
culture, politics, and health for centuries. It's often instructive to consider an issue through the lens of connections
with tobacco. One such issue is: who takes responsibility for
what?

Working at the National Center for Health Services
Research, I asked a secretary if she would photocopy
one page for me. Her curt reply was, "That's not in my job
description." She had clarity about her role and was not
about to deviate from it. In contrast, one day as Syracuse
Dean I returned to my office to find my thoroughly reliable
administrative assistant, Marcia Wisehoon, missing without
note or explanation. Later, I learned this: A call had come
from frantic parents whose son had been struggling with
depression and had expressed suicidal ideation. He had not
answered or returned their calls, and they had just heard he
missed his Health Services appointment. Marcia located the
son's roommate, who had seen him moments earlier in the
student center. She immediately went there, found him, and
personally delivered him to psychiatric care. That was not in
her job description, but she may have saved his life.

When David Kessler led the Food and Drug Administration, he knew smoking was a leading cause of prevent-
able death and serious illness. He lacked legislative authority
to regulate the lethal drug nicotine or the toxic additives in
cigarettes. He did have jurisdiction over medical devices, so
he classified cigarettes as drug delivery devices and issued

regulations limiting their use and promotion. Sued by the tobacco industry, he lost. But the process of discovery in that trial revealed incriminating evidence that company executives knowingly strove to addict young smokers in order to create future markets. Some of those executives were later criminally prosecuted and convicted. Although Kessler lost in court, he won a major public opinion victory which accelerated the cultural transformation that has radically reduced the prevalence of smoking, severely constrained where it can be done, eliminated most of its promotion, and saved untold millions of lives. By not accepting the limitations of his job description, Kessler acted outside the scope of his role. We are in his debt for that.

We each occupy many roles:—in our work, neighborhoods, families, and many more. Each role has expectations and constraints, often in conflict with one another. We can't avoid deciding when to accept and when to transgress those constraints and expectations. In the Covid era, medical personnel have been torn between the desperate need to help patients and the obligation to protect and care for family—and their heroism resides in their deciding to place themselves in harm's way for a larger purpose than their personal interests. How we make those choices reveals our character and values as clearly as anything can.

Some folks approach a closed door aware that another person follows, and they hold the door open for that next person. Others just go through without such regard. I think of the former as Wake Watchers and the later as Obliviods. I have observed this difference on campuses, in airports, hospitals, and stores—wherever there are doors. I have no hypothesis about what accounts for this difference. For some people it may be a stable pattern of behavior; for others it may vary by occasion. A similar difference shows up in the behavior of smokers. Some are sensitive to the sensitivities of others; some are oblivious or indifferent.

As a new assistant professor at Western Reserve University (soon to join Case Institute of Technology to create Case Western Reserve; see Chapter 16), I was unsure how to deal with a full professor whose pipe seemed more a part of him than just something he held. Whenever it went out, he relit it. He even did that when we were in a small elevator. I wanted to shriek about his failure to wait even a moment until we reached our floor, but I knew that my fate was also in his hands. I left the elevator at the next floor and continued up the stairs. His tobacco wasn't the only thing burning.

I brooded and bided my time. At the next department meeting, he was, as always, smoking the pipe. It was an unusually cold, windy February day. I opened one window wide, and then another. The temperature in the room plummeted. He protested. I replied that I didn't mind the cold at all. In fact, I found it refreshing, given how severely his pipe smoke was clouding the room. He set his pipe aside and detente ensued. I closed the windows, and the problem did not recur.

The appearance of sensitivity to others can be hypocritical: an illusion, a perilous trap. At the request of a senior development officer, I joined her on a visit to the program director of a private foundation that supported higher education. She understood, as good fundraisers do, that donors support people they know and trust more than programs they have been told about. They like to hear directly from those who will do the work, not just from someone boasting about how great the work will be. When we entered the officer's elegant office, he greeted us warmly, pulled a cigarette out, and said "Do you mind if I smoke?" I thanked him emphatically for the kindness of his question and said I would much prefer it if

he did not. He put the cigarette away. The development officer looked daggers at me, later scolded me, and never again
asked me to go on a development call!

Now, decades later, no such question would likely arise.
The evolution of cultural practices around smoking has
transformed the experiences of smokers, the smoke-averse,
and policymakers. There's more needed; for example, drivers must have children properly secured in approved safety
seats but are free to fill the car with toxic fumes, gassing the
children as they go. But overall, the progress is heartening.
Therein lies the reason for optimism. With imagination, a
willingness to take risks, and tenacity, we're waging an
encouraging battle against the harms of smoking. And we'll
eventually win it, even if we must do that two pipes, two cigarettes, and one cigar at a time.

SMOOTS, FRATS, AND GRAPES

Even after someone stops drinking, alcohol in the stomach and intestine continues to enter the bloodstream, impairing judgment and coordination for hours.

—The JED Foundation, 2023

The bridge over the Charles River on Massachusetts Avenue from Boston to Cambridge is 364.4 smoots long, plus or minus an ear. Many metrics are used to measure length, such as feet, meters, angstrom units, light years, inches, or miles. To measure, one needs a measuring instrument, e.g., a yardstick, calipers, surveyor's wheel, or micrometer. The instrument must be accurate enough for the purpose: a cheap yardstick might work for deciding how much driveway sealer you need, but not for ordering living room drapes. And you must know how to use the instrument properly.

Oliver Smoot was a pledge at the Lambda Chi Alpha fraternity at MIT. Some clever lads there decided that, at 5' 7", he could be both a metric and a measuring instrument. A smoot was defined as a distance equal to his height, and he was the instrument for measuring. In October 1958, at the Boston end of the bridge, he stretched out on the sidewalk. A line was marked at the Cambridge end of him, and he then moved or was moved one smoot to that point. The process was repeated across the bridge; the length to the other end was 364.4 smoots, plus or minus an ear. This event—the subject of articles, books, commemorations, and lectures—is woven into the fabric of MIT's identity and is among the most famous examples of MIT's tradition of pranks, known there as "hacks"—a usage unrelated to computer hacking. When Protagoras of Abdera said "Man is the measure of all things" in the fifth century BCE, he prompted millennia of deliberation about what he meant. I am confident he did not mean smoots.

In my first year at MIT, I walked across that bridge countless times going from the Pi Lambda Phi fraternity in Boston to the campus. That was two years before the smoot markings. Every Friday we had an examination from 9 to 10 a.m. in one of the required courses, always in the same room, furnished with drafting tables rather than desks. The subject rotated among physics, chemistry, and mathematics. In a nightmare, I had studied for a physics exam only to find that our exam that week was in chemistry. I mentioned this to classmates and learned that many others had comparable anxieties, terrors, and dreams. One guy studied so late that, as dawn approached, he thought it folly to sleep for the few remaining hours. He went to the exam room early and put his gear on the drafting table. Then, with time to spare, he went to the men's room. He awakened abruptly, on the toilet, at 10:30, having missed the exam. Some of us had learned that being well-rested was more prudent than any amount of study; others never learned that lesson.

I joined a fraternity because I had met and liked some of its members, the food was vastly better than in the dormitories, and being in a supportive community of reasonable size was appealing. Many members had awe-inspiring minds and irresistible wit. Several have had lustrous careers not only in engineering and the sciences, but in law, medicine, architecture, film production, and more. There were some fine moments. The older students were typically generous in helping younger students academically, about anything ranging from a specific homework problem to choosing courses for a subsequent semester. And there was plenty of good-natured wit along with an abundance of unpredictable pranks.

Yet, I had misgivings from the start. The rituals of pledging, hazing, and initiation were pretentious, absurd, demeaning, and dangerous. I endured them with unexpressed disdain. As a member, I was even less comfortable; it was one thing to undergo such nonsense, a worse thing to be complicitly inflicting it on others. And although some of the parties were majestic (one involving dazzling decorations was covered by the news media) the focus on alcohol was abhorrent. The last straw was when the house hired a buxom stripper, whom some of the inebriated members were gleefully groping. I soon resigned from the fraternity.

MIT cleaned up its fraternity practices long ago. A detailed policy makes it a serious offense to perform any act of hazing, however subtle, and even to be aware of such acts and fail to intervene or to report them. But despite decades of national effort, hazing, drunkenness, and misogyny remain widespread elsewhere, especially among predominantly white fraternities, causing harm so severe that in 2021 fifteen students at Washington State University were indicted for not intervening in a hazing ritual that caused the death by acute alcohol intoxication of nineteen-year-old pledge Samuel Martinez at Alpha Tau Omega. Six students at Bowling Green University were charged with manslaughter after a similar incident killed Stone Foltz at Pi Kappa Alpha. University leaders rail against these episodes of death by alcohol, yet themselves often validate drinking as the modal way to celebrate. Thus, my thirty-fifth year at Syracuse University brought a gift from the chancellor—a pair of crystal wine goblets from Tiffany and Co. I don't use them.

Notwithstanding imprudent excursions into reckless debauchery, the fraternity mostly maintained the sobriety necessary for academic survival. MIT was and is a profoundly serious place. Study time could be somber, with occasional disruptive bursts of wit. One mainly taciturn classmate mastered material with otherworldly ease and had an almost perfect record in each course. In our sophomore year, he entered the room where I was studying, leapt into the air, fired at me with a cap gun, and on his way out said, "That was a jump shot." After MIT he went to Harvard Medical School. Without their knowledge or consent, he enrolled simultaneously in a master's program at MIT in electrical engineering. He explained that to me later as "a strategy to keep his mind alive while he endured the tedium of pre-clinical medical school."

Another member was editor of *VooDoo*, the venerable campus humor magazine. The cover of one issue reproduced a faculty parking permit. The day after that appeared, few faculty could park in the lot; it was nearly filled with student cars displaying the replica, which had duped the lot's attendant. MIT has published three books about its tradition of imaginative hacks; the *VooDoo* prank was not included. I inquired, and learned it was excluded for violating the Code of Ethics that governs hacks. One principle of that Code is that pranks must "not damage anyone, either physically, mentally, or emotionally." They must do no harm to persons or property. The book editors decided that harm was done to faculty whose parking expectations were thwarted, and perhaps to students whose faculty showed up late. The *VooDoo* editor became a research scientist of great accomplishment and acclaim as well as an exemplary teacher.

Whether a stunt did harm requires clarifying what its consequences were and then assessing their severity. It's not like measuring the smoots across a bridge. One might try to compile a list of prohibited actions, but creative hackers will always be able to contrive stunts that aren't on that list. Unlike the extensive and detailed policy prohibiting hazing, the Code of Ethics for hacks states just a few very general principles. The acceptability of a hack will be judged by standards, not rules, in Kahneman's terms.

The minimum age for drinking alcohol during my college days was twenty-one. That was statutory: unambiguous, requiring no judgment or interpretation. Without enforcement, the statute was irrelevant. Fraudulent IDs were unnecessary. The fraternity had a liquor dealer in Brookline who provided whatever was wanted without asking about the ultimate consumers. Authorities also turned a blind eye to underage drinking. Even the most raucous bacchanalia drew no official attention. That was reserved for serious matters, like obstructive parking. On one such evening I heard a police loudspeaker announce: "Warning, all cars triple parked on Beacon Street must be moved immediately or they will be towed." A few people scrambled toward the door.

Just as it's useful to consider issues as they relate to tobacco, it's instructive to look through the lens of relationships to alcohol. In my teens I learned to enjoy wine, and to respect moderation, when it was served by my parents or their friends in homes or restaurants. My taxonomy was simple: wine not good enough to drink, acceptable wine, good wine, and great wine. My early experience parallels that of many young people in other countries, such as France. American students sometimes drink, and encourage others to drink, to get drunk. I had a student from France, in a class of twenty-five, who expressed mystification at this attitude. She said that in France they drink wine because they love the wine. If they drink too much, as sometimes happens, that's an unintended and unwelcome effect. She added that when she first overheard an American student say, "Let's go get drunk tonight," she could not understand what was happening, because it seemed so obviously foolish, ill-considered, and immature. If I had made this point in class, I doubt it would have influenced the students. But when their French class-mate did so, they seemed to recognize a new perspective as enlightening and perhaps, for some, a sobering conversation.

The statutory definition of inebriation is typically a blood alcohol content (BAC) of .08 percent or more. An instrument—the breathalyzer—measures breath alcohol content in connection with police apprehensions for suspected driving under the influence of alcohol (DUI). Breathalyzer results are usually accepted as a reliable surrogate for BAC, allowing a prosecutor to infer the BAC from those results. Some jurisdictions have eliminated the inference by making the breathalyzer result sufficient grounds for conviction. So there's a metric and an instrument. However, whether or not a driver is stopped on suspicion of DUI is not regulated by any algorithm; it's exactly the kind of decision that can be influenced by bias, the circumstances of the officer on that occasion, and the patterns of behavior characteristic of that officer. Even if these distortions were eliminated, there remains prosecutorial discretion—where inconsistencies of many kinds abound.

Between the Western border of New York State and Erie, Pennsylvania, a repaved stretch of Interstate 90 has a speed limit of 55 mph. For much of that stretch, if you drive at 65 cars will zoom past you, sometimes with noticeable annoyance. In residential neighborhoods where the limit is 35, you won't likely be stopped at 38, but at 45 you're asking for trouble. If you want to see the ghost ships of Mallows Bay in Maryland, you must cross the Quantico Marine Base. The speed limit there, mostly 30 mph, was recently lowered to 20 or even 15 in some parts. Drive even a few miles too fast and you'll likely be apprehended. Don't mess with the Marines.

In any jurisdiction the decision about how strictly to enforce speed limits is political. It can be corrupt, discriminatory, designed to increase income from fines, sensitive to contextual factors such as weather conditions, or fashioned to serve the public interest. However such decisions are made, they will be made by people making judgments. The best protection against bad judgment is transparency with accountability, so that all stakeholders can understand and advocate based on accurate information. The best provision for good judgment is training decision makers, as Kahneman et al. advocate, in what processes can minimize flawed choices. Eliminating judgment altogether is a hopeless fantasy.

Judgmental fallibility is inherent when human behavior is involved. The length of a bridge, the speed of a car, the level of alcohol can all be measured with appropriate degrees of precision. Determining what degree of precision is appropriate can't be measured by any instrument, nor can determining what policy best serves the interests of a given community. Human affairs proceed by an interplay of facts and values, clouded often by poor evaluation of evidence, inconsistency of goals, and cognitive biases. We can always strive to do better, advancing one smoot at a time.

MARCHES, MAJORS, MONITORS, AND 1862

... the building is the kind of academic melting pot that gives university presidents indigestion.

—Alex Beam, *The Boston Globe* (October 30, 1996)

ROTC was mandatory for first- and second-year students when I entered MIT in 1956. For reasons I don't recall, I chose the army. I learned to take an M-1 rifle apart, clean it, and reassemble it. I learned what the army considered competent shoe shining and brass polishing. I learned to read maps. That's about all. I was dreadful at drill and dozed in dimly lit rooms at lectures with projected slides and a narrative I thought suitable for the sixth grade at most. I got bad grades.

MIT was chartered by Massachusetts on April 10, 1861, but had no funds for operation. Two days later the Civil War began at Fort Sumter. The Morrill Land Grant College Act was signed into law by Abraham Lincoln on July 2, 1862. Lincoln's commitment to education was especially impressive considering that he was at war. MIT's founder, William Barton Rogers, was able to secure Morrill Grant support in 1863, and MIT opened its doors in 1865 with a focus on agriculture as part of its mission. We had to take ROTC because MIT was a land grant university under the provisions of that support. There was no distinction between public and private universities then. Today, all colleges and universities supported by the Morrill Act are public except for MIT and parts of Cornell. MIT still offers ROTC, but it's no longer mandatory.

In 1861, Lincoln had recently commissioned the ironclad warship USS *Monitor* as part of the war effort. It was built in Brooklyn, NY, launched in January 1862, fought the Battle of Hampton Roads in March, and sank during a storm and disappeared in December 1862. Lincoln paid a personal visit to the hospital to see its surviving captain. Subsequent ships of like kind were known as *Monitor*-class warships.

Despite my unhappy time in ROTC, I decided, ambivalently, to continue beyond the required years. The Vietnam War was developing ominously, I was disinclined to be a draft dodger, and I assumed that being a commissioned officer was better than being a drafted foot soldier. Continuing in ROTC required an application and interview. A skeptical Army Major, noting my poor record, asked why I aspired to stay in the program. I didn't mention the war or the draft but said I had heard that the advanced years of the program respected the intelligence of the cadets and that the prior years convinced me that the Army was in serious need of intelligent officers. Nonetheless, I was admitted to the program. I began my third year still marching, and now getting a stipend of 90 cents a day for being in the advanced program. I was better at marching in a straight line on the drill field, however, than through the MIT curriculum. That was more of a Brownian walk, as I took courses that did not cohere into any recognized major. When the new major in Humanities and Science was introduced, it opened a supportive path for me. I had to choose one technical field and one humanities field; I picked mathematics and philosophy. That fostered my desire to aim for a graduate degree in philosophy. But my commitment to ROTC was in the way. I went to the ROTC office in Building 20 to say I wanted to withdraw from ROTC. The conversation was something like this:

Sergeant, loudly erupting: "You can't do that; you made a commitment. There's a contract. We have it in writing. There's no way you can quit. Why would you want to drop out?"

Student: "I've decided to go to graduate school in philosophy."

Sergeant, incredulous: "Philosophy? *PHILOSOPHY??* OK, you can quit."

So we processed the paperwork. I returned my uniform, except for the khaki shirt. I was out, but checks kept coming. I asked that they be stopped, and eventually they were. I had received several unearned checks, however. At 90 cents a day, it didn't amount to much, but it was the army's money, so I took the checks back. The irascible sergeant said, "Kid, you've caused us enough trouble already. Cash the damn checks and don't ever come back."

ROTC wasn't alone in Building 20. If a building can be the soul of a university, Building 20 was that for MIT. A drafty, temporary wartime structure built in 1943, it was expected to last just a few post-war months. But universities always cherish any available space, and one thing after another went into Building 20 as it became a beloved wonderland of diversity and innovation for the next fifty-five years. It was home to the MIT model railroad club, to a bunch of brainstorming physicists (nine of whom ultimately won Nobel Prizes), to the first office of Noam Chomsky (who was creating the field of contemporary linguistics), to the first research on loudspeakers by Ambrose Bose. And it housed the lab where Harold (Doc) Edgerton was inventing stroboscopic photography. Edgerton soon became known as "Papa Flash," but that did not reflect the range of his creativity. He was constantly inventing new ways of seeing and doing things—and that takes us back to 1862.

Some oceanographers had despaired of finding the long-lost USS *Monitor*; others held hope of success. In 1973 an expedition from the Duke Marine Lab hunted where others had not thought to look. Supported by the expedition ship's crew, eight scientists conducted the search. To great international acclaim, they found USS *Monitor* on August 27, 1973. The oldest of the scientists was Edgerton, then 70, using his side-scan sonar for the first time in an underwater venture. The youngest scientist was Cathryn Newton, then a 16-year-old Duke sophomore. Decades later she became my associate dean of arts and sciences at Syracuse, then the dean, and my co-author on several research projects. Thus she, too, is part of the lineage of MIT and Building 20.

I wore that khaki shirt in graduate school when painting furniture or walls. It accumulated splotches of various hues and became my regular painting shirt. I use it still; by now it's a palimpsest sixty years in the making. Our minds are like that, too, accumulating layers and hues that stay with us, sometimes blending, sometimes fading, sometimes reminding us of past actions or perceptions we can use in new creative ways. When I see that shirt, I think of its early days and also of the tremendous respect I have gained since then for many military leaders and for the values and traditions they embody. I also think of Building 20 and the indomitable spirit of creative energy it inspired and continues to inspire in all who have the good fortune to be part of its legacy.

13

TITLES, COPS, AND MILKSHAKES

I've thought of various titles such as Bank Night in Hollywood, Sutter's Last Stand, The Golden Peepshow, All It Needs is Elephants, The Hotshop Handicap, Where Vaudeville Went it Died, *and rot like that. But nothing that smacks you in the kisser. By the way, would you convey my compliments to the purist who reads your proofs and tell him or her that I write in a sort of broken-down patois which is something like the way a Swiss waiter talks, and that when I split an infinitive, God damnit, I split it so it will stay split.*

—Raymond Chandler, letter to *Atlantic Monthly*
Editor Edward Weeks (January 18, 1947)

Books have titles, as do reports, lectures, and people. Choosing them and using them mixes opportunity and peril, because people care greatly about these ever-present labels. When the New York State Task Force on Life and the Law held a twentieth Anniversary Symposium at Rockefeller University on March 3, 2005, my address to them was called *Talking about Titles*. I said that I'd had a longstanding interest in titles because of my early academic experience. I was a graduate student when Michael Dummett, visiting from Oxford, gave a talk titled "Bringing About the Past," in which he argued that in principle it should be possible to influence what had happened earlier. I thought that had to be wrong and realized that the perfect title for a rejoinder would be "Leaving the Past Alone." I really wanted to use that title; I worked on a response for about six months, and (with Dummett's generous help) it became my first publication. I couldn't bear to see that title go to waste.

Titles can prompt vigorous dispute, laden with emotion. In 1976 I was invited to speak at UC-Irvine. I proposed "Moral Mayhem in Modern Medicine" to provoke and intrigue, not to inflame and not especially to inform. But what a fuss ensued! After an oddly long silence, my gracious host phoned and awkwardly, diplomatically, said what amounted to this: "We can't say that in Orange County. It could offend the local medical community in ways we can't afford. Please change it." I changed "Mayhem" to "Muddles" and gave the same talk I had intended to give, adding a commentary about their sensitivity to the original title.

I wrote a book titled *Doctors' Dilemmas*, published in 1982. That title was chosen, over my objections, to placate a lunatic editor. The manuscript for *Doctors' Dilemmas* had the working title *Doctors of Virtue*, with the subtitle *Moral Conflict and Medical Care*. "How clever," I'd thought. "We want physicians to be virtuous as well as competent. Moral philosophers study virtue, and this book is about the relationship between them, hence, the richly ambiguous *Doctors of Virtue*." My editor said, "The subtitle's okay, but you'll have to change the title. "We can't sell a book with the word '*virtue*' in the title." (Alasdair Macintyre's masterful book *After Virtue* was published in 1981 to sustained national acclaim.)

"Okay," I said, "what should I call it?"

"We can't tell you," she replied. "It's your book. Something punchy."

"Punchy?" I asked. "What's that?—A technical term in publishing? Give me an example."

"Well," she answered, "we sold six million copies of *Jonathan Livingston Seagull*."

"Fine," I said. "So, call it *Samuel Gorovitz Penguin*."

"You're not taking the problem seriously," she complained.

"Everyone I've asked likes the title I had," I replied in defense.

"They're irrelevant," she explained. "Titles aren't for the people you interact with. They're for browsers. The judgment of the people in your circle doesn't matter."

"But," I whimpered, "*I* am in that circle, so how can I pick the title?"

"Something really catchy," she persisted, "but with some relation to the content."

"Okay," I proposed, "how about *The Hourly Orgasm Weight Loss Plan?*"

"You're still not taking the problem seriously," she scolded.

I gave up.

Once, I imprudently agreed to give a talk over a year in advance at a meeting on ethical issues in forensic psychiatry. I had no idea what I would discuss. With about six months to go I was suddenly asked for a title immediately. I sent this: "Could Oliver Wendell Holmes, Jr. and Sigmund Freud Work

Together if Socrates Were Watching?" I wrote that to be vague, create an illusion of content, and buy time. The meeting organizer loved it, apparently not realizing that all it meant was that I would say something or other probably within the general area of the conference.

Titles like that wouldn't do for the Task Force. We needed the titles of our reports to have clarity, content, and gravitas. The Task Force had its own breed of title examiners, not concerned with real estate but with real communicative effectiveness. Given my special interest in titles, I became the informal title generator for our reports. Thus, when we wrote a report about proxy decision-making, the proposals for a title sounded approximately like this:

"Ethical and Legal Aspects of Making Health Related Decisions for Persons Who Lack the Capacity to Decide on their Own Behalf."

I said, "No. Let's call it 'When Others Must Choose.'" And they did.

Then, when we considered physician-assisted suicide, the proposed titles sounded like this: "The Strengths and Weaknesses of the Various Arguments for and against the Proposition that New York State Should Modify its Legal Prohibition against Assisted Suicide."

I said, "No. Let's call it 'When Death is Sought.'" And they did.

I was on a roll as Task Force Titlemeister. But I was summarily fired from that role after the sordid matter of the report on reproduction. We wrote a large volume on the use of medical technology in assisting those whose more-standard efforts to have children were unsuccessful.

I said, "Let's call it 'Love's Labors Lost.'"

Thus ended my career as Chief Title Guy. They wanted fresh material, not something already used.

While based throughout at Syracuse, I had eight or nine full or part-time, or visiting, sometimes overlapping, appointments at various other places. Understandably, people were confused about what titles to attach to me. When the Task Force used one I had shed a year earlier, I reported this to Tia Powell, the executive director. She'd clearly had more than enough fussing from me, and proposed to simplify matters henceforth by giving me a special Task Force title: Grand Vizier and Celestial Ark. I liked Celestial Ark especially, and thus considered Tia to be the new Task Force Titlemeister.

Once my book appeared, I was on the book tour treadmill. Some interviews went well, and I learned surprising things from the process. In Los Angeles, I took a taxi to the studio for a morning program on CBS. I was scheduled for about five minutes "between the peanut butter lady and Hodding Carter." Moments before the program a producer came to the greenroom and said my segment was cancelled because local bookstores did not yet have my book, adding that viewers expect any book they discuss to be available. I asked for a brief reprieve, called my publisher in New York, unleashed some language I will not repeat here, was assured that the books would be in Los Angeles stores the next day, presented my case to the producer, and was back on the schedule. When my turn came, a slick, polished interviewer asked questions the producers had prepared for him. He had no apparent awareness of the content of the book beyond the notes he was given. As soon as the commercial break between segments began, he was gone. I then asked one of the staff how to get a taxi to my hotel.

Staff: "A taxi? You didn't come in a limo? You could have had a limo. Why didn't you come in a limo?"

Me: "My hotel is a mile away. I didn't need a limo to take me a mile. I just want a taxi."

Staff (to Other Staff): "This guy didn't come in a limo. He wants a taxi. Anyone here know how to get a taxi?"

Other Staff: "No idea. Try the newsroom. They might know."

They did; a few minutes later I was at the hotel.

The session with Larry King could not have been more different. It was an hour long, including commercial breaks. A studio light indicated on or off the air. When the light turned red, King did not leave. He continued the conversation with keen interest, referring to specific passages of the text. He cared about the issues in a smart and probing way. It was a privilege to have that encounter, especially when off the air. (That interview was later rebroadcast within "The Best of Larry King.") Studs Terkel, too, was a joy. His well-read copy of the book had marginalia, highlights, many corners turned down, and notes inserted in various places. He knew the content and cared about it.

And in 1982, there was *PBS Latenight*, originating in Detroit and carried by 80 PBS stations. The host, Dennis Wholey, was thoughtful and engaged with the material. Several times he spoke directly to the camera, holding a copy of the book and referring to "our guest" as the author of the new book *The Doctor's Dilemma*. I was astounded, but being young and naive, I let it pass, every time. Although he had the book in hand and in view, he never perceived the title accurately as *Doctors' Dilemmas*. (On later occasions, when others did that, I had the maturity to reply, "I am a great admirer of George Bernard Shaw, who wrote *The Doctor's Dilemma*, but I am not George Bernard Shaw and did not write *The Doctor's Dilemma*. I wrote *Doctors' Dilemmas*, which is our subject today.") I could not fathom how Wholey could make such a perceptual mistake, unable to see what was right before him, thinking he was seeing what was familiar and expected.

Among my strongest recollections of that otherwise excellent interview was that I had said hospital patients should prepare written lists of all their questions and should insist that attending physicians sit down at the bedside to talk with them, rather than stand over them, accentuating the tremendous imbalance of power that already distorts doctor-patient communications. And I recall learning from the station, a few days later, that they had many complaints from physicians about how that interview made it much harder for them to complete their rounds.

So I thought.

The station had given me a studio recording of the interview, which I rediscovered in 2021 on a large and obsolete tape format I wasn't sure there was any way to view. There was: a professional service copied it to a DVD. I watched it. Some of what I remembered was true. Wholey did botch the book title, every time. But the story about patients writing their questions and delaying the doctors was not my story! It's a story Wholey told to support what I was saying, in his comments about an earlier program. I must have preferred my version so much that I believed it, false though it was. More revealing is that in the interview I wanted to mention, as an example, the premature birth of a 469-gram baby. As far as I know, no one heard what I actually said, revealed to me only as I watched the recording. I leapt from my chair in horror as I heard myself cite the case of a 469-pound baby. *Ouch!*

That kind of misleading perceptual auto-correct, ever-present, is often innocuous but can be extremely danger-ous. Here's an example. I was alone at home when a sudden explosion of sound shattered the tranquility. The doorbell rang with rapid-fire repetition along with frantic pounding. I opened the door to find a distraught and disheveled woman, a bundle of trembling terror and tears. The bucolic street was on a favorite route for runners and walkers; she was just passing an adjacent wooded area when a man had jumped out of the woods, sexually assaulted her, and fled in his car. A moment or two later I had given her the toothbrush and toothpaste she requested, called the police, and set a lawn chair in the driveway for her. The police came swiftly and treated the woman with kindness and respect. Of the four, three were white, one Black. The Black officer was at the roadside, the others in the driveway. The victim was on the lawn chair; from the garage, I could overhear the conversation as she told her story and responded to questions. A white cop asked if the assailant was Black or white. She said she did not know, but she saw his car as he drove away, and the car was black. The cop then said to another cop, about 30 feet up the driveway, "She said the guy was Black." I rushed up to the Black cop and reported what I had heard. He sighed and said, "Every day, man. Every day." The attacker was caught and went to prison. He was white. There was a good outcome in this case, yet legions of innocent Black men are booked and sometimes even convicted because of errors like the one made by the cop in my driveway.

But back to booking of a better kind! Here, too, the law plays a role. Copyright law protects intellectual property, much as patent law protects inventions. Copyright for the content of a book may be assigned to the publisher, the author, or a third party such as an estate or survivor, and it can be transferred from one to another by agreement. But book titles have no protection. Anyone can use any title for any book. I could do a book entitled *The King James Bible Revised for the Twenty-First Century* and put it on a book that claimed milkshakes were good for one's spiritual state and then contained only recipes for milkshakes. Given the gullibility of the market for printed junk, it might sell well at airport stalls or supermarket checkout displays.

I did not know titles were unprotected when in 1991 I obtained the copyright for my book about Boston's Beth Israel Hospital. I had no serious title battles with editors that time, just a minor skirmish when I was told the word "philosopher" could not be in the title. Oxford University Press was content with *Drawing the Line*. The subtitle was *Life, Death, and Ethical Choices in an American Hospital*. Four years after my book appeared, another Syracuse University professor published a book also titled *Drawing the Line*. The author, Mark Monmonier, is a renowned cultural geographer; his subtitle was *Tales of Maps and Cartocontroversy*. In this elegant book, Mark reveals the perils of assuming that maps provide credible information. Each map tells the story its maker wants to convey. Boundaries depicted in a map may be no more than an effort to persuade the viewer that those boundaries are real and should be respected. He writes:

> As powerful tools of persuasion in science and public affairs, maps have had a remarkable effect on our view of the world, our health, and the impact of our votes. At the root of their power is our frequently unquestioning acceptance of cartographic messages . . . like other artists, map authors select what suits them and ignore what doesn't. Militant informed skepticism is the citizen's best defense against cartographic harassment by bureaucrats or ideologues.

How we organize domains of interest is also a kind of mapping: science here but art over there; law in one place and emotion in another. Those boundaries are illusory; Mark's Message, like Wiener's Warning, sharpens our thinking and helps protect us against being deceived by our own artifacts.

As the stories above reveal, the titles of books can be among the last items resolved. The Dummett story shows that a title can be embraced first, prompting the work that follows later. And titles can vary in different markets, such as Darwin's *On the Origin of Species,* which for the American market unfortunately lost its crucially important "On."

Because thinking about titles can stimulate thinking about content, at the Task Force Symposium I charged the participants to speculate about what future titles might be. Although actual titles are chosen only after reports are finished, contemplating what they might be could provide a rich sense of the Task Force's future—bleak if it weren't possible to imagine what later reports might be about. As examples, I suggested: "Proper Preparation for Pandemic's Pandemonium"; "Will the Task Force Lose Face if It Doesn't Consider Face Transplants?"; and "Can We Stem the Tide of Conflict about Stem Cells?" The participants offered many ideas, and some of the subjects were later addressed. We did a report in 2015 on guidelines for pandemics and tried to assist when Covid struck in 2019 by offering to collaborate in managing the rapidly emerging crisis. We were rebuffed by Andrew Cuomo's administration, but that's a different story. (Were I to write it, I'd title it something like "Paranoia, Arrogance, and Micro-managing." Or maybe, "Delusional Entitlement vs. the Public Interest.")

The stories I did choose for this book have titles that could only be written at the end, because although I chose the stories, I could not predict where any of them would go once the telling began. After each was drafted and revised many times, I could then see what it had to say and seek terms that might pique your interest and prompt you to read on. I'm grateful that you've read this far.

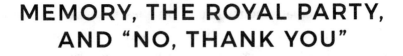

MEMORY, THE ROYAL PARTY,
AND "NO, THANK YOU"

Recollection, I have found, is usually about half invention.

—Wallace Stegner, *Crossing to Safety* (1987)

Studies of memory showed long ago that the vividness and specificity with which we recall an event and our intense confidence in that memory are unreliable evidence. Some of what we're sure we remember can be proven never to have happened. Some of what we're confident never happened can be proven to have been important events in our lives. That's why Katharine Whitehorn's autobiography, *Selective Memory*, bears an appropriate and honest title. She writes:

> Sherlock Holmes refused to remember things
> he thought of no importance, of no use to him;
> but not many of us can order our minds so

neatly. The memory makes its own selections, its own decisions about what is fun, interesting, moving, or even excruciating to remember, and what is simply too boring to store. What's more, you can remember things that didn't happen—and you aren't lying, either. The brain apparently sees thing A and thing C, and if it is puzzled by the gap, officiously fills in what it thinks should be there, thing B; then you remember that, and when you've recalled it two or three times it's a genuine memory— but of the last time you ran this construct past your consciousness.

Digging around among old papers and letters, as I have been, I was occasionally staggered to see just how wrong my memory of something could be. To guard against such false memories, Katharine resolved to work as if she were doing a biography of someone else—examining such primary sources as contemporaneous newspaper accounts and archival records, interviewing witnesses, and consulting other relevant records. As a student at Cambridge University, she had kept in touch with her deaf mother as well as possible. Her mother could not use the phone, so Katharine sent letters frequently. After her mother's death she found a cache of those letters; she was unaware that her mother had saved them. There, she discovered—in her own hand—accounts of important events she would have claimed never happened but for this compelling evidence.

This is not disclosed in her book; I know it only because Katharine, a friend and colleague, explained her research process to me. (It informed my approach to this book. I am using all available resources to minimize errors from false memories.) Katharine and I started working together after meeting at a health policy conference in Europe—perhaps at WHO in Geneva, but my memory fails on that—and I soon learned that she was a unique and pioneering force in British journalism. By example and by the power of her prose and presence, she had an elevating influence on opportunities for women, quality of health care, practices of cooking, parenting, and much more, even including the design of airports. I once asked a visitor from England if he knew of her, and he leaned forward and replied, "*Every* literate Briton knows Katharine Whitehorn."

Katharine had spent much time in the U.S. and had friends and contacts here long before I knew her. In 1991 she came to work on a piece on feminist issues, and I gladly helped her with some logistics and by setting up connections with a few people she didn't know. Her appreciation seemed out of proportion to that small amount of help so eagerly provided. During her visit I also hosted a dinner for the visiting Peruvian writer Mario Vargas Llosa (later to win the Nobel Prize) and, to her great delight, sat Katharine next to Mario.

Katharine's husband Gavin Lyall, a man of many talents and a prominent writer of thrillers (what we call mysteries), kept his own quiet counsel and did not travel with Katharine on her professional trips. She was exuberantly extroverted; he was sweetly gracious to visitors but showed little interest in the many social events to which she was called. So in 1994 Katharine asked me to be her companion at a black-tie event at the Royal Society of Medicine, explaining that Gavin would be profoundly grateful to me for getting him off the hook and she was sure I'd enjoy hearing the Irish psychiatrist Anthony Clare. It was a grand event.

Two years later Katharine asked me to attend an Inaugural Professorial Lecture at Westminster University by another eminent psychiatrist, Patrick Pietroni. I was puzzled by her unusual instructions, directing me to bring my passport and arrive at a precise moment. Entering was akin to going through airport security because, as I learned on arrival, the lecture would be given "in the presence of HRH The Prince of Wales." Katharine led me to our seats near the stage. The first row was empty. Once the audience was settled, the Rector, Dr. Geoffrey Copland, asked us to rise for the Royal Party. Prince Charles and his entourage took seats in front of us. After the lecture, we were again asked to rise and remain in place until the Royal Party had left. There would then be a buffet lunch and reception for the audience in a large hall on the main level. As the Royal Party headed out, Katharine tugged on my shoulder. Resisting and puzzled, I said, "We're told to stay here until the Royal Party has left." Sternly, she replied, "Oh, don't be difficult. We're *in* that." And off we scrambled to a balcony where about two dozen people, including Prince Charles, had gathered.

Katharine, who seemed to know everyone, introduced me to the Rector and Prof. Pietroni, then walked away. As we chatted briefly, I saw Prince Charles talking with others some distance away. The next thing I knew, Katharine arrived with Prince Charles in tow, introduced us, took hold of the Rector and Professor Pietroni and with a firm grip on each, marched them away—leaving me suddenly alone with Prince Charles. Later, she confessed that the entire caper was contrived as a thank-you for her 1991 visit to Central New York!

The British obsession with formalized protocols about titles is familiar. I knew, from working on the PBS animated documentary *Castle*—based on David Macaulay's 1977 book—that the title Prince of Wales has been conferred on the (male) heir apparent to the British throne since the fourteenth century. When one met Charles, the Prince of Wales, one was first to call him *Your Royal Highness* and, thereafter, simply *Sir*. But I saw none of that. He greeted me with a warm smile and ready handshake, and we began to talk. I was instantly mindful of the difference between what we think and what we say. Among my simultaneous thoughts was "Oh, your tailor is SO MUCH better than mine!"—he was a paragon of sartorial elegance to the finest detail. And "The tabloids portray you as merely a knave and fool. I don't believe that. I'm eager for this glimpse of what you really are." I said no such things. We talked about the importance of holistic approaches to health, about doctor-patient communication, about modernism and architecture. And I thought, "You might sometimes deserve bad press. But whatever else is true, you really are a thoughtful, serious, and pretty smart guy."

A server arrived with beautiful hors d'oeuvres on a silver tray. I said I'd already tried them, and they were excellent, but Charles thanked the server and politely declined. He then explained that he may make more than a dozen ceremonial appearances in a single day. In defense, his strict policy is to decline all refreshments—a strategy for survival. Ever since, I have thought of that as "Doing a Prince Charles," and am often much the better for emulating it. After we talked for six or seven minutes, one of Charles's aides came (with Katharine's permission, I assume) to move him to the next stop in what I saw as a highly programed, demanding, and constraining marathon. He has now assumed a far more challenging role.

When we move to a new role, we bring ourselves into it. However, that new role also changes us, sometimes for the better and sometimes for the worse. And the sense we have of ourselves—of our values, experiences, strengths, and weaknesses—is based largely on the memories, true and false, that we carry about ourselves. What we do in our roles, old or new, depends on who and what we think we are. We relate variously to the roles we occupy—filling them with distinction, or relinquishing, redefining, overstepping, or even renouncing them, as Queen Elizabeth's uncle Edward did when he left the British throne in 1936, and as Charles's son Harry has recently done by saying "No, thank you" to the Royal Family and shedding his princely entitlements and burdens. Such wrenching separations result from the tension between personal relationship roles and professional or lineage roles. We all fill multiple roles at all times, so tensions about which role should dominate when they conflict are ever-present. It need not be about relinquishing a throne; health care providers in the Covid era face agonizing daily conflict between professional commitments and family responsibilities. Even episodic tensions can be anguishing, as between showing up as expected to see a child in a school performance or attending a sudden, unexpected and important meeting with a client or donor. The apologetic parent who "makes it up" to that disappointed child with a grand outing the following weekend perhaps is unaware that the outing may not erase a hurt that can linger and lurk across the years.

Whatever we do makes memories for ourselves and nearly always for others. As Katharine explained, those of us who are not Sherlock Holmes have limited control over what we remember and how accurately. When we make memories for others, we can strive to do well by them and hope we have created good memories that the people we care most about will later select fondly.

FACES, FAME, AND FIRING

I've learned that bitterness gives you wrinkles.

—Rosanne Cash, *NPR TED Talk* (August 31, 2022)

As our memories shape our sense of who and what we are, so do our faces. Often, we recognize those we know in other ways—how they move, their silhouette, a distinctive hat—but it is by the face that we most commonly recognize others and how we are commonly recognized by others. Who does what with our images can alter our lives. New NCAA policies—and court decisions—allow high-profile college athletes to share in the profits from commercial uses of their names and images.

Facial-recognition software is used increasingly for law enforcement and for political suppression of dissident views, and facial images can be constructed or altered by sophisticated software. These developments raise concerns about protecting privacy and about discriminatory software that is less accurate in identifying persons with darker skin than those typically white skins used as illustrative in the training of dermatologists. This leads to more false positive identifications of people already disadvantaged in other ways, such as by poverty, living in neighborhoods with unhealthy environments or poor access to health care, or being women, or having a disability. Pictures of people, however made, typically include images of their faces even when they are not portraits. And that presents the recurrent challenge of seeing beyond appearances to the underlying reality, which might be entirely different depending on the actual life circumstances of the persons whose images we see.

As far back as the sixth grade, I had a darkroom. Fascinated by photography, I've taken thousands of pictures of architecture, shadows, nature, and people ever since. Long ago I realized that any person "smiling for the camera"—(whether told to or not)—looks inauthentic. The best portraits often have no smile. Of those that do, we know at a glance whether the smile is genuine. Unless we are trained actors, we cannot voluntarily activate the facial muscles that express genuine laughter or happiness. When I want subjects to look cheerful, rather than thoughtful, troubled, or absorbed—the trick is not to tell them to smile, but just to be funny and capture the involuntary smile. The same applies to laughter; one who laughs intentionally to appear amused does not look like one whose laughter stems from amusement. (Some people's facial movement characteristics are different; they may be unable to smile or may have unusual involuntary facial movements.)

Reading what's revealed in a face is a skill, imperfect as is any empirically based judgment. Paul Ekman, the famed psychologist at the University of California at Berkeley, is the most prominent scientific investigator of decoding micro expressions—brief, tiny, involuntary facial movements that are triggered by our thoughts and emotions. His work is widely influential and also controversial. But it has established at least that what is on our minds and in our hearts shows up to some extent on our faces. And wherever we go, our faces go with us.

How we have lived also leaves its imprint. The skin of a long-time smoker, a sunworshipper, a ranch hand, or a foundry laborer will show the accumulated imprint of gradual changes across the years. And the person who is chronically negative and contrarian, who repeatedly is "a sourpuss," may acquire a sour puss. That's what Abraham Lincoln understood. A familiar story about Lincoln recounts his refusal to appoint someone nominated for his cabinet. Asked why, he allegedly said, "I don't like his face." When the candidate's advocate exclaimed that the man bore no responsibility for his face, Lincoln asserted, "Every man over forty is responsible for his face."

Because facial images affect people's lives profoundly, even the ability to recognize someone provides a power that can be used for good or ill. And discrimination against those with facial differences is a severe and generally unacknowledged barrier to their inclusion. For example, the highly talented Canadian singer Ani Spooner tells of the moment when she was performing at a night club before a group of enthusiastic fans when the owner of the club arrived, saw her for the first time, and fired her on the spot because he did not want his customers to have to look at a singer with a port wine disfigurement on her face. She subsequently founded the "About Face" project and is a leading advocate of understanding, acceptance, and inclusion based on each person's merits, rather than merely on appearance.

Karen Metzler was born in 1951 with spina bifida and multiple other medical problems including facial disfigurement. Treating her aggressively, her medical team beat the odds and she survived. I met her through a pediatrician in Cleveland when she was still a student. Having great intelligence and awe-inspiring tenacity, she later earned a B.A. from Baldwin-Wallace College, magna cum laude (1974), and then an MSSA from Case Western Reserve's School of Applied Social Sciences (1984). Karen had much she wanted to say, and I agreed to present her case to the students in a bioethics class at CWRU. Initially, I only described her dire neonatal circumstances. The students vigorously debated the ethics of treating her aggressively. Some weeks later I said we would return to that debate, this time with an expert guest. Karen then entered the classroom, slowly, on crutches because of the amputation of a leg. What Karen most wanted was for the students to speak their minds candidly, knowing that this might require courage on their part. I recall most clearly that when a student asked whether, given her many impairments, she thought the decision to save her was right, she said, "It depends on when you ask me. Some days yes, some days no." A slightly edited transcript of what she said that day (in *Moral Problems in Medicine*, pp. 458-463) included these comments:

> I wanted to be strong, to be healthy. But most of all, I wanted to be accepted by others. And it appeared to me that the rules were that in order to be accepted, I had to keep to myself any of the negative aspects of being handicapped, because society had to deny them

in order for society to be free of discomfort. I am taking, now, a big risk in being honest and open about my feelings and perceptions, which means that I do not sugar-coat any which may need it for social acceptability . . . . Am I less human as a person because my body is not like that of other humans? Are my feelings, thoughts, needs, and desires different from theirs because my body is? . . . . it is my hope, then, that I have enabled you to feel more comfortable and willing to deal with the emotions surrounding handicappedness for both sides.

A few years later, at Maryland, I invited Karen to meet with another class. She came to College Park and the visit was equally successful. Later, at one of the finer traditional French restaurants nearby, Karen seemed enthralled. Then, suddenly, a dark cloud seemed to pass over her. She leaned forward, and teary-eyed, said, "I appreciate this so very much. No one has ever taken me to a restaurant before." I was grateful to learn of that aspect of her experience.

By the time she was forty, Karen had earned national stature as an author, speaker, and advocate for the disabled. She had long since accepted her facial characteristics as part of her unique human identity and strove tirelessly to encourage each person to value the unique identity of all others.

Lincoln did not have Karen Metzler in mind when making his comment about people earning their faces. But he had ample reason to make a more limited claim about earning one's face, because he already knew what war inflicts. In 1861 at the Battle of Fredericksburg, Oliver Dart Jr. was struck by shrapnel and lost much of the lower right quarter of his face. The National Archives contains a photo taken on December 13, 1862, showing the extensive damage. And on May 3, 1863, at the Battle of Chancellorsville, Private Joseph Harvey was hit by a shell fragment that destroyed much of the right side of his face. A photograph of the result is at the National Museum of Civil War Medicine in Frederick, MD. In Lincoln's time, facial disfigurement and other disabilities were prevalent.

Here are three anecdotes about recognition: (1) With no internet connection on my cell phone in Sitka, Alaska, I approached the public library to see if I could send an email from there. A young man I didn't recognize welcomed me at the door, saying, "Professor Gorovitz, can I assist you?" (2) After landing at LaGuardia Airport, washing my hands in the men's room, I heard a lad at the next basin say, approximately, "Hiya, Professor Gorovitz! Howya doon'?" (3) On a bridge to Canada, the toll collector greeted me by name.

Having taught thousands of students over six decades, I understand that one will recognize me occasionally. Each time, it surprises and pleases me. But I am no celebrity. Wondering how being readily recognized might feel to genuine celebrities, I asked my friend and colleague Rock Brynner about his famous father's experiences. Rock had written of Yul Brynner's traumatizing horror in confronting autograph seekers after performances of *The King and I*:

> Frank's [Sinatra] mean streaks, like my father's, seemed to me justified by his unique stature as an artist. Traveling with either of them, what one experienced was an aggressive if

well-meaning public that could suddenly swell into a turbulent crowd jabbing out at eye level with pens and other sharp objects. When situations became genuinely menacing, they were not easily forgotten. Frank and Yul were both young men when they required cops on horseback at the stage door nightly; the hateful view of strangers which that fosters helps to make celebrity a slow-acting poison . . . Psychologically, the relentless attention of complete strangers is abnormal, and gradually induces a state of perpetual self-consciousness . . .

Stage-door effects thus ripple into daily life. Celebrities are also seen in restaurants, shops, and parks. Rock said, "For forty years, Yul was immediately recognized everywhere he went all over the world. There's no simple answer to how he reacted. It depended on the context, on the behavior of the fans." Much as he relished stardom, his celebrity created presented an ever-present burden. (With hindsight, we can recognize that *The King and I* has offensive misogynistic themes and exploits racial stereotypes. It was, nonetheless, among the most widely seen musical theater shows and movies throughout the world.) Actor and author Nick Offerman makes a point that parallels what Rock related (*Where the Deer and The Antelope Play*, 2021):

One truly wonderful silver lining about the pandemic has been the freedom that masks have given me to pass in public undetected. There are many instances which can have their tone completely altered when people recognize me.

Few faces are known throughout the world. But social media now make images of millions of faces available on request, all over the world. Artificial intelligence already offers the possibility of rapidly gathering images of someone else, as reported by the *New York Times* (May 26, 2022):

> You upload a photo of a face, check a box agreeing to the terms of service and then get a grid of photos of faces deemed similar, with links to where they appear on the internet. *The New York Times* used PimEyes [a photo-finding app] on the faces of a dozen *Times* journalists, with their consent, to test its powers . . . PimEyes found photos of every person, some that the journalists had never seen before . . . PimEyes found one reporter dancing at an art museum event a decade ago, and . . . a photo that she didn't particularly like but that the photographer had decided to use to advertise his business on Yelp. A tech reporter's younger self was spotted in an awkward crush of fans at the Coachella music festival in 2011. A foreign correspondent appeared . . . in the blurry background of a photo taken of someone else at a Greek airport in 2019.

It may be possible to submit the cell phone image of a stranger, along with the question, "Who is this?" and get an identification—accurate or not—in reply. Law enforcement agencies may already have such capacities. If the algorithms of identification reflect the same kinds of biases that infect police eyewitness lineups, anyone concerned with justice should worry. The Museum of Lost Memories uses social media to circulate photographic images of unidentified people and sometimes can confirm an identity with help from among its vast numbers of followers. Further, two unrelated people can look almost indistinguishably alike, as epidemiologist Tim Spector, of King's College in London, has shown by using facial recognition software to identify doppelganger strangers: unrelated people resembling each other enough to be taken for identical twins. He has found many such pairs. False identifications can happen for other reasons, of course. In November 2021 the French police arrested Khaled Aedh Al-Otaibi for the murder of American journalist Jamal Khashoggi. On December 8, they released him, admitting it was a different person with the same name they were seeking. Had they looked carefully at his passport they would have known it was a misidentification. It is unclear whether Inspector Clouseau was involved.

No great painting can be seen properly in haste. What one sees evolves as one looks into the painting, and such a wealth of detail can't be grasped casually. Rembrandt's *The Night Watch*, in the Rijksmuseum in Amsterdam, is inexhaustibly fascinating. Painted in 1642, it's among the world's most acclaimed and studied works. Massive, at approximately twelve feet high and fourteen feet wide, it contains about twenty faces, each of which merits analysis and interpretation. As I gazed intently at one of them, a young woman approached and said, "Please excuse me for interrupting. But I can't help asking. Are you Sam Gorovitz?" This wasn't a former student; she had not seen me before. But she and her husband, a classmate of my son's, had recently visited him. A keen observer, she noticed the photographs in his apartment and remembered the faces. In Amsterdam, she thought I looked familiar enough to prompt her inquiry.

People often do resemble one another. That's not just a concern for eyewitness testimony, it's been a problem for me. Some folks have claimed that I look like Bernie Sanders (I don't), like Gene Wilder (I can see that), like Larry David (it's true), and sometimes that I look to them like people I don't resemble at all. In August 2022, as I walked past a house with unusually appealing landscaping, I turned to express appreciation to the homeowner tending to it. She was a retired art teacher I'd not met or seen before, and as I was about to speak, she said, "You look like Frank Lloyd Wright." I'd not heard that one before; I asked whether she meant how he used to look or like how he looks now. That might be a disputed point.

During the intermission at a concert, someone I'd known for years told me he greatly enjoyed my recent presentation at the Thursday Morning Round Table in Syracuse. The rest of the conversation went like this:

> I: I've been to Thursday Round Table meetings, but not recently. I've not done any presentations there.
>
> He: Yes, you have. I saw you.
>
> I: What did I talk about?
>
> He: The role of the U.S. State Department in International Negotiations. You were excellent.
>
> I: Oh. Well, that's a topic Ambassador Goodwin

Cooke would have addressed.

He: Yes. That's what you talked about.

I: I've known Goodie Cooke for years. I admire him greatly. But I never have been Goodwin Cooke.

He: Of course you are.

At that point I stopped arguing about whether I was myself or someone else and staggered back to my seat for the rest of the concert.

My confidence in my identity had not been shaken. Yet it was a stark reminder that actions can be attributed to me based on a false perception of my identity. The result might not be unwarranted praise. It could be inconvenience, embarrassment, or even indictment and the most severe consequences of criminal conviction. Recognition, like memory, can be accurate or erroneous. When we are accurately identified, or taken for someone we are not, that can help or harm us. We must confront these connected issues. If we do, in the spirit of Lincoln's perspective, perhaps in forty years we'll look as though we've done it well.

In 2021 my cousin Debbie Berg and her husband planned a hiking trip in Olympia National Park in Washington State. They wisely arranged for a professional guide (I'll call him EK) to optimize their learning, the experience of the natural environment, and safety. Over the five days they spent together, the conversation with EK turned from time to time to their families, interests, and backgrounds. When EK mentioned attending Syracuse University, my cousin asked, "It's a large university, I know, so this is unlikely. But did you ever hear of a Professor Sam Gorovitz?" By her account, EK stopped short and, wide-eyed, asked "Sam Gorovitz? Do you know him?" She replied, "He's my cousin," at which point, she reports, he "nearly fell off the mountain." EK had been in my class, which, he said, "in one day changed my life." He referenced a story I told in an introductory ethics course in 2001 about a letter I received from an alumnus. The gist of that letter was this: "In my final semester I cheated on my calculus final. I was sure I'd be fine, because no one would ever know. But I was wrong. I know, and I have known ever since, and I can't take it anymore." This is an example of what Daniel Pink calls moral regret (in *The Power of Regret*, 2022), which, as Pink notes, can exert its power far into the future.

What we remember about ourselves, as noted earlier, helps shape our sense of who and what we are. As we evolve over the years, the effects of that sense can also change and sometimes surprise us. The events in our minds are real events, with real effects. In 1992 Syracuse University faced a severe budget crisis. The trustees mandated a pernicious plan that protected their favored Newhouse (Communications) and Maxwell (Public Administration) schools from deep cuts imposed on the rest of the university. No one wanted to eliminate faculty positions, but it wasn't clear that could be avoided. The vice chancellor instructed the deans to make provisional plans in case such draconian measures were necessary. At a deans' meeting, he directed us to identify, confidentially, the order in which untenured assistant professors would be fired.

Typically, I take careful notes at serious meetings. Many people doodle when bored. I'm doodle-challenged, so I don't do that. Nor do I write poetry. (Poetry is extremely hard; my colleague Mary Karr has written eloquently of what it takes to create a fine poem, describing one she worked on for two years before its sixtieth draft appeared in *The New Yorker*.) My coping mechanism is doggerel, a far less demanding and comparatively frivolous form of expression. Here's what I scribbled during that meeting; these are essentially my notes from December 8, 1992:

> 12/8/92 Academic Deans Cabinet
>
> "Fire the youngsters" the VC proclaimed.
>
> "Fire the slow and the weak and the maimed."
>
> "That's how our budget distress is relieved."
>
> (Okay if later a few are reprieved.)
>
> "Set the priorities! Reallocate!"
>
> (Guidelines will follow at some later date.)
>
> "And when we've made changes all over SU
>
> We'll think up the reasons to which they are due."
>
> "Then after we think all the danger is done
>
> We'll all be invited to share in the fun
>
> Of a strategy game that's dropped in our laps
>
> Because of some newly found financial gaps."
>
> And what are the values that guide all the fuss?
>
> We're told that they're basically all up to us
>
> As long as in detail they strictly conform
>
> To each centrally chosen forthcoming norm.
>
> (These notes reflect the insensitivity of the times;
>
> no such satire would be acceptable today.)

After that meeting, I rejected his directive, making three points to him. First, I acknowledged that I served at his pleasure and that if he did not rescind his directive I would resign as dean immediately. Second, I explained a basic flaw in his reasoning by invoking his love of classical music. I was negotiating then with many senior professors who were contemplating retirement, some of whom were open to considering deals that might be to mutual advantage. Those negotiations were still pending. I asked him to envision an orchestra conductor being told to identify the most expendable musician, while management was negotiating possible retirements among the percussionists and violinists. How could you know whom it would be most damaging to lose, I asked, without knowing which sections will be most depleted for other reasons? He accepted my argument and dropped his demand.

But the third point was perhaps the most important, so I pressed on. It appeared to him that if we did not inform the untenured faculty of a secret expendability list, no harm would follow. He was wrong. Had I designated any assistant professor as most expendable, perhaps because of perceiving that professor as having some weakness or deficiency, that designation, even unexpressed, would have consequences. I would thereafter think differently about that person; that young professor would have a diminished standing in my mind, and that would be a harm. Like the alumnus who had cheated on his calculus exam, I would know, and that knowledge could be corrosive. I might not choose that person to serve on an important committee or for a multi-year research initiative, for example. Fortunately, the vice-chancellor's doubly flawed scheme was terminated, no assistant professors were targeted, and in the end, all were retained, untainted, when retirements yielded enough to meet the mandated budget goals.

Decades ago, I heard that a London newspaper printed a scathing letter insulting the author of a recent book. Hurt and mystified by the attack from someone who had been a friend and supporter, that book author wondered how it could possibly be. Then the newspaper, with apology and embarrassment, printed a retraction admitting that the letter had been attributed to the wrong writer. One might expect this disclosure to dispel both the mystery and the resulting hurt and anger. Not necessarily. I discussed this with the ever-insightful Katharine Whitehorn, who observed that as the book author pondered how that attack could have happened, he may have had ideas about the possibility. An author with a vivid imagination could conjure all sorts of speculations: for example, the book author could have imagined the letter writer wrongly suspecting a dalliance between his own wife and the book author. If I now think a bad action is possible by someone I previously thought incapable of it, my view of him has changed. I may think less of him and act less confidently in respect to him. My mind has been primed to be more suspicious. In reconsidering his possible behaviors, events have occurred in my mind, real events with consequences, as would have happened if I had targeted untenured professors without letting them know.

What we are told influences what we think. Our thoughts are not entirely within our control. Recall the effect of someone telling you not to envision an elephant! When we are told that we are, or seem to be, a specific person, we cannot help but process that claim, one way or another. An event with real effects takes place in our minds, and because those effects can benefit or harm us it matters whether what is said about who we are is accurate.

Discerning the difference between appearance and reality is a traditional goal of philosophical inquiry: investigating the gap between how things seem and how they are. Another tradition, which philosophy shares with the sciences, is to identify the assumptions being made and examine the quality of evidence that supports those assumptions. The scrupulous investigator does not make claims beyond what the evidence supports. A classic story of rigorous adherence to the highest standards of evidence involves the renowned Ernest Nagel of Columbia University. According to legend, he was walking along when an accident occurred in an intersection in front of him. One of the cars sped away. Later, as a witness in court, Nagel was asked, "Was the car you saw leaving the scene a blue car?' And his maximally careful reply: "The side of the car I saw was blue."

The facial recognition conundrum brings Nagel's concerns to the fore. Am I who I seem to be, or is that a misperception by someone else? Are you who you seem to me to be, or am I seeing someone else you strongly resemble? Am I justified in claiming I saw you, or ought I say, "The side of the face I saw looked like you?"

I'm more cautious now when I think I recognize someone; who they seem to be at first glance has sometimes been shown by closer inspection to be a misperception. I'm grateful that I am who I seemed to be to my former student, EK, who served my cousins so well in Olympia National Park. He's the same former student who greeted me by name at the library in Sitka many years earlier! For me, he's achieved some fame of his own. He's led a life of cherishing nature, educating others to appreciate and protect it, serving both his clients and the natural world with kindness and caring. I've reconnected with him and see that, now over forty, he has earned a face that Lincoln would admire.

MERGERS, MURDERS, AND A HAT RACK

Murder most foul, as in the best it is / But this most foul, strange and unnatural.

—William Shakespeare, *Hamlet* (1603)

Mergers—joining independent entities into one—are messy and risky. Some fail spectacularly, like the merger of the Stanford University hospital and the University of California Medical Center at San Francisco in 1997. It cost $79 million to initiate the merger and millions more to disentangle it when within two years it was a demonstrable failure. That story is told candidly in the Winter 2000 issue of *Stanford Magazine*: "The venture's biggest downfall may have been that it never managed to bind the two institutions together with a common culture. Most professors continued to identify almost exclusively with their home campus." And " . . . integrating computer systems at the two schools cost $126 million, five times what was expected. 1,000 employees were brought on board after the merger. Proponents of the venture had projected only 200 new hires." Prediction is common; accurate prediction is rare.

Marriages also are mergers, with unimpressive success rates. Estimates vary, but by all accounts, nearly half the marriages in the U.S. end in divorce or separation, with divorce rates higher for second marriages and higher still for third. Larry King, such a charming interviewer (as noted above), married eight times; his marriages lasted for periods from a few months to more than twenty years. His was a prodigious talent, but he was no master of marital mergers. He brought charm, excitement, celebrity and wealth into these relationships, but he didn't bring durability. In addition to bringing their backgrounds, affections, attributes, and expectations into a marriage, a couple also brings their stuff. That may include cars, pets, stuffed animals, photos, and all sorts of other things. And books.

During the eight years Anne Fadiman spent writing her classic *The Spirit Catches You and You Fall Down*, she wrote occasional essays about books and how book lovers relate to them. Those essays are collected in *Ex Libris*, which begins with an eight-page account of two people bringing their book collections together. Anne and her husband, also a writer and book lover, had been together six years. Each had a substantial library with considerable overlap between them. To create a single library, do they keep the pristine copy, the dog-eared annotated copy, or both? Should the books be arranged by subject matter, chronology, or otherwise? Do books inscribed by the author have a special place? Each question yields deep inquiry, illuminating far more than topics about books. As we grapple with the questions, we consider the values that attract us to or repel us from each possible answer. We recognize the conceptual connections among the ideas the question raises. We wrestle with our own ambivalence and consider what compromises we are willing to make, and why. After reading those few Fadiman pages eight or ten times, I was still learning from them. The essay's title: "Marrying Libraries."

Just as two hospital systems can each have their own group of pediatricians or radiologists, and two libraries can have their own sets of work by Dickens, two universities can each have their own set of physicists, parking guards, and accountants. In 1964 I became an assistant professor at Western Reserve University, adjacent to Case Institute of Technology. The famous Michelson-Morley experiment in 1887, among the most significant in modern physics, was a collaboration between the physicist Albert Michelson at Case Institute of Technology and the chemist Edward Morley at Western Reserve University, whose labs were just steps apart. That work led to Michelson's Nobel Prize in physics in 1907, as the first American to win a Nobel in the sciences. Over the decades, there were many examples of cooperation between faculty at the two schools, and at times even talk about more formal association. But nothing came of that until the 1960s, when Western Reserve President John Millis and Case President Keith Glennan agreed that federation would create a university of greater national distinction. They established a study commission of national leaders in higher education and public policy, charged with exploring the idea. The Heald Commission, chaired by former Ford Foundation President Henry Heald, in its "Vision of a University" report, predicted that federation could create a premier private university.

In 1967, Case Institute of Technology, with its emphasis on engineering and science, and Western Reserve University, with professional and liberal arts programs, formed Case Western Reserve University. The idea of merger was anathema; the plan was to create a single institution with two semi-autonomous parts. I was there at the creation. The first problem was that no one wanted to give up anything. People are heavily invested in names, in what those things they care about are called, be they book titles, Task Force reports, personal roles, or institutions. Dispute about a name for the new university arose at the outset. Some people advocated calling it the University of Cleveland, citing the University of Chicago as an exemplar of excellence. But Case folks complained that it did not contain the name Case, and Western Reserve folks objected that it erased the name Western Reserve. Some even expressed an embarrassing elitist fear that it might invite a misperception of the university as public rather than private, and therefore less worthy of admiration. So, Case Western Reserve it is. I've never found anyone who considers that a graceful or convenient name.

The two schools did few things alike. Their academic calendars differed, as did their fringe benefit plans and even that supremely important matter of access to parking. One faculty proposal urged that for each item among the fringe benefits, the new university should adopt whichever of the two plans was more generous. That would have been prohibitively expensive, so the administration developed compromises. A dependent tuition benefit at WRU paid for one degree per dependent. (A colleague who later worked for me as a pre-med advisor waived the right to have his daughter's college tuition covered; he won that bet when she used the benefit later for a free medical degree.) At a meeting called to explain the proposed benefit compromises, a professor from Case said, "I know the tuition benefit covers one degree per child for any number of children. Does it also cover one degree per spouse?"

The planners had not anticipated that question; I wondered whether any current spouses were equally surprised.

Glennan, proudly a Republican who had been NASA's first administrator, was a distinguished engineer with substantial industrial experience before becoming president at Case. He retired from that position in 1966 once the federation was launched. John Schoff Millis was also an accomplished scientist, but his trajectory was entirely academic. He came to WRU from the presidency of the University of Vermont. Millis was an unwavering advocate of inclusion and equality. He built a strong physics department by hiring superb physicists who had been victims of the McCarthy investigations, holding that scientific quality should be the sole basis for appointment decisions, not unsubstantiated allegations about their politics or even substantiated claims that they had expressed dissenting political views. Glennan and Millis led very different tribes when they each stepped aside for the appointment of CWRU's first president, Robert Morse.

Tribal cultures are long-lived. To understand the chaos and despair that beset Lebanon today, one must consider the lingering influence of four hundred years of Berber history. Those who attributed Covid vaccine resistance in African American communities to suspicions borne of the unconscionable Tuskegee experiments overlook an understanding, centuries old, that enslaved persons and their descendants could be abused as research subjects with impunity, and the Tuskegee horrors were just one more unsurprising example. And some historians of science have suggested that Einsteinian physics became accepted not by persuading traditionalists, but when enough of them finally retired or died to shift the culture to the more open perspectives of younger scientists.

Morse was a distinguished physicist with superb credentials in academia and government. He had been dean of the college at Brown after chairing their physics department, and then assistant secretary for research and development in the Navy. He left that post because of his displeasure with the war in Vietnam, with which he did not want to be complicit. He became the last president of Case in 1966 and the first of CWRU in 1967. Little did he suspect what explosive events would await him. Protests against the war in Vietnam were already widespread on campuses across the country. CWRU was a hotbed of anti-war leadership, with prominent anti-war pediatrician Benjamin Spock on our faculty. He had campaigned for Lyndon Johnson in 1964, fearing that the hawkish Barry Goldwater was too dangerous, and assured by Johnson's pledge not to escalate the war. But Johnson did escalate, and Spock's sense of betrayal and outrage was white hot. I met with him and others almost weekly to discuss opposition strategies. Protests at CWRU were sometimes joined by supporters from afar, such as young Jack Nicholson and Candice Bergen. Spock retired from the faculty in 1967, and in a testimonial banquet on May 29 it was said that "he has helped our children differentiate between truth and falsehood." Nobel Laureate and Medical School Dean Fred Robbins spoke at that event, as did Coretta Scott King. Although that ended Spock's presence at CWRU, the protest strategy group continued seething about the war. Satirist Tom Lehrer came to Cleveland to help support anti-war candidates; he and I put on fund-raising events in some homes in the area. A performance by Lehrer brought people in; I did the pitch for funding. (Nicholson, Bergen, my linguistics teacher Noam Chomsky, and Lehrer, much older now, at this writing in 2022 are still supporting the values that brought them to the protest.)

My physics colleague Jonathan Reichert and I chartered an old DC3 (N144A) and organized a group trip to an anti-war rally and to hear Martin Luther King, Jr. at the United

Nations Plaza in New York on April 15, 1967. New York City Police estimated the crowd at 125,000. Ben Spock joined King among the protest leaders, and King explicitly linked protesting the Vietnam war with protests supporting social justice in the United States. He stressed that the disadvantaged poor—black, brown, white, or anything else—should have common cause with one another:

> I believe everyone has a duty to be in both the civil rights and peace movements; but for those who presently choose but one, I would hope they will finally come to see the moral roots common to both. I hope they will understand that brotherhood is indivisible, that equality of races is connected with the equality of nations in a single harmonious co-existence of all human beings . . .

> We are arrogant in professing to be concerned about the freedom of foreign nations while not setting our own house in order. Many of our senators and congressmen vote joyously to appropriate billions of dollars for war in Vietnam, and these same senators and congressmen vote loudly against a fair housing bill to make it possible for a Negro veteran of Vietnam to purchase a decent home. We arm Negro soldiers to kill on foreign battlefields, but offer little protection for their relatives from beatings and killings in our own South . . .

> Let us save our national honor—STOP THE BOMBING.

I would like to urge students from colleges all over the nation to use this summer and coming summers educating and organizing communities across the nation against the war. I have already talked with students who are organizing in this vein from such schools as Harvard University on the banks of the Charles River in Massachusetts and my own Morehouse College in the red hills of Georgia. We must all speak out in a multitude of voices against this most cruel and senseless war. The thunder of our voices will be the only sound stronger than the blast of bombs and the clamor of war hysteria.

In 1968 other protest leaders, including Chomsky, stopped in Cleveland en route to the Democratic Convention in Chicago. The Chicago Police Riots there led to the prosecution in 1969 of the Chicago Eight (later the Chicago Seven), the subject of much attention including a recent documentary film. (Julius Hoffman, the presiding judge, behaved so outrageously that all the convictions decided by the jury and the resultant sentencing were vacated on appeal in 1972.) King's plea was still unheeded; the bombing had not stopped. In Spring 1970, Nixon launched a blistering military assault on Cambodia with even more bombing. Protests immediately erupted across the nation. For many, that was the final straw, and at Kent State University the most aggressive activists intensified their disruptive behaviors, leaving King's plea for nonviolence also unheeded. Knowing this history is necessary for understanding what happened there in 1970.

On May 4, 1970, Ohio National Guard soldiers, acting at the behest of Governor James Rhodes, murdered four unarmed Kent State students. The protest was not merely expressing dissenting views but was disruptive of normal campus operations. That disruption could certainly have been handled in non-lethal ways, but the dissenting views were anathema to Rhodes and his ilk. One of the murdered four was not even protesting—just walking to class.

These murders became international news within hours; Mississippi state police killed two Black students at Jackson State College on May 14; that gained less attention. A national commission concluded later that the police action there "was an unreasonable, unjustified overreaction."

Some mergers are planned; others just happen. Kent State, only about forty miles from Cleveland, closed immediately after those murders. Many of their students then made their way, somehow, to Cleveland, merging with thousands of protesting CWRU students blocking Euclid Avenue—the main street by Severance Hall, home of the Cleveland Orchestra—thus creating an incendiary standoff. As dean of CWRU's Adelbert College (established October 26, 1882), I was the guy in the street going back and forth alone, between the Director of Public Safety and, behind him, mounted cops with their badges obscured, eager to bash student heads, and the intransigent protesters blocking the street—trying to negotiate a nonviolent way to defuse the conflict. The DPS agreed to hold back his massed forces briefly. And the students listened, moving to the sidewalks, reopening the road.

CWRU remained troubled, with protesters occupying the hallways of the main administration building, Adelbert Hall—the same building that was dedicated in 1882—as university leaders strove to navigate a safe passage through exams to commencement. Rather than adopting Governor Rhodes' approach of lethal force, CWRU's President Morse, Provost Herman Stein, and Assistant Vice-President Ernie Green engaged the protesting students with coffee and doughnuts, attentive listening, honesty, and sympathetic understanding even where there was firm disagreement. They averted tragic disaster that day and in the following weeks, but there was no averting trouble. The students occupying the building addressed their "demands" to Morse. He had already publicly called the war poisonous, yet some protest leaders aimed their rage directly at him. One tried to break into his office by running toward the office door, using a floor-standing hat rack as a battering ram to break the lock. Standing by to defend that door, Green, a former NFL All-Pro star, calmly snatched the front end of the speeding rack—stopping it as if it had hit a brick wall and twisting it so sharply that the student clutching the other end was spun off the floor and launched, airborne, into submission.

The nation's leading baroque music ensemble, the New York Pro Musica, was in residence at CWRU that week, scheduled to play on May 5 in the beautiful gothic Harkness Chapel. Noah Greenberg, the founder (1952) and director of the ensemble, had died in 1966 and was succeeded by John Reeves White. But White was unable to make the trip to Cleveland, so the group was "rudderless" according to Shelley Gruskin, then and still a legendary master of the baroque recorder. In a recent conversation, he recounted vivid memories of a long, tense meeting of the group on the evening of the 4th. All the musicians opposed the war, appalled by the killings and supportive of the students' cause. LaNoue Davenport, their director of instruments, moderated the meeting and advocated canceling the concert on the grounds that "business as usual" was inappropriate in the face of such outrages. Shelley favored reframing the concert as a memorial to the murdered students. He recalls the meeting as contentious and distressing, leading to a vote to reframe and present the concert. Davenport accepted that result.

The soprano Elizabeth Humes also has vivid memories. Speaking to me from her seaside home in southern France, she recently said she does not remember clearly what happened—who said or did what—but she does recall how she felt. "I was absolutely horror struck that government would do that. How is it possible? I thought, whatever we can do to help we ought to do. I have a fundamental memory of wanting to do what we could, of asking what we could give. It was a crushing feeling. I felt we must do the concert. And it was not just a concert, that feeling of being crushed lingered for days." Although none of us is clear about the particulars, we all think it likely that LaNoue explained to the audience that the concert was a memorial to the murdered students and that they should listen in silence and without applause at any point. My own clear memory is of the visual beauty and musical perfection of that candle-lit concert—as beautiful and moving a ceremony as any of us had experienced—and of an emotional impact that defies description.

Mergers can also change the character of a participant completely and abruptly, with dreadful consequences. Boeing Aircraft was among the world's most admired and trusted companies before it merged with MacDonald Douglas. The Boeing culture had honored safety as the highest priority, with respect for the insights and talents of its engineering and manufacturing employees. Boeing had bought MacDonald Douglas, whose executives then outmaneuvered the Boeing leadership and gained control. As soon as they did, maximizing the price of the stock became the overriding objective, the Boeing "no shortcuts" culture was replaced by a culture of deception and concealment, and the flawed 737 Max was aggressively marketed with more than 5000 sold. The company internally knew it was unsafe; two planes crashed, and hundreds of people died as a result. My MIT classmate Rob Stengel, a leading expert on flight dynamics, provides a definitive analysis of the basic facts that doomed those flights at http://www.stengel.mycpanel.princeton.edu/737MAX.pdf.

We have found in earlier chapters that viewing topics through an atypical lens, such as relationship to tobacco, alcohol, or learning English, can help us see in a new and useful way. When the lens we adopt is the concept of mergers, we are prompted to ask ourselves new questions. First, it is not clear what counts as a merger, so we might ask, "Is this situation I am in, or am considering, even an example of a merger?" Or is it just a juxtaposition, an interaction? Many cases are clear one way or the other. But what about meeting a friend for coffee, getting onto a crowded bus, flowing with other parents into a PTA meeting? If we view such situations as mergers, and think about why mergers succeed or fail, we may think and act differently even in those situations.

Some mergers, like the California hospital example, last briefly. Some are extremely short, like the marriage of Irish singer Sinead O'Connor to Barry Herridge—which lasted somewhere between 7 and 16 days, according to various accounts. Some mergers last for millennia: the Ucayali and Marañón rivers flow together to form the Amazon River. Is there a minimum duration for something to count as a merger?

Mergers are most likely to thrive when the merging entities have a symbiotic relationship, each providing something importantly supportive of the other. Lichens were long seen as ideal exemplars of such symbiosis, with algae and fungal filaments (mycorrhizal networks) interacting to create stable organisms with properties neither had alone. That's an oversimplification; we've learned that the creation and functioning of lichen involve complex interactions among extensive networks of many players. Yet some marriages do seem, similarly, more like mergers between large and complex familial corporations than like the deliberate choice of two autonomous, mutually attracted individuals! Whatever circumstances bring us into interaction with other individuals or groups, if we think about mergers and what enables them to thrive—like the Pro Musica musicians whose only thought was, "How can we help?"—we may be more inclined to consider what we can contribute than merely to focus on what we can gain. And that seems a lesson worth learning.

17

MENTORING, A DOG, AND A SHIPWRECK

"A ship's a being in its own right, like a person, so to speak, that thinks, and breathes, and reacts."

—Jacques Yonnet, *Paris Noir: The Secret History of a City* (1954), translated by Christine Donougher (2006). This passage was spoken by the "dangerous thief" named Keep-on-Dancin'.

My senior thesis adviser at MIT, Abner Shimony, was just ten years older than I. He was calm, gentle, and terrifying. I'd already revised my draft several times, addressing his incisive critical reactions. We met in his small office to discuss the latest version. He agreed it was clearly better as he returned the pages covered with new criticisms. Seeing my fear and disappointment, he continued, "I know. It's hard. But we want the best you can do. You can still improve it.

I'm going through the same struggles with my dissertation adviser." I was mystified.

Already an MIT professor with a philosophy Ph.D. from Yale, he explained that he was completing his doctorate in physics at Princeton with the legendary Eugene Wigner (you met Wigner in Chapter 2), who insisted Shimony's work be the best it could be. Learning this, I saw Shimony's unrelenting scrutiny of my work as the most respectful gift he could give me. And I realized that philosophy and physics blended in his mind in ways that enabled him to see more deeply into each. The next year, I was also a Ph.D. student. My Stanford classmates agonized about the academic demands. As I breezed through, my view of Shimony evolved from deeply appreciative to reverential. Ever since, as student, professor, and administrator, I have been guided and inspired by that paradigm of mentoring excellence.

In addition to rigor, good mentoring is attuned to the passage of time. Some of my peers gave dissertation drafts to their advisors and heard nothing for months. Such discouraging delays corrode confidence and prevent progress. My dissertation advisor, David Nivison, was an exemplar of ideal support. This soft-spoken, Lincolnesque specialist in Chinese philosophy would receive my draft and return it with extensive, thoughtful comments in a matter of days, sometimes even bringing it to my door on his way home. People have often asked how I could complete a doctorate in record time; a crucial ingredient was Nivison's spectacular mentoring.

David Nivison died in 2014 at 92. Patrick Suppes, another important mentor for me, for whom I was a teaching assistant, also died in 2014 at 92. Abner Shimony died in 2015, just 87. Nivison and Suppes were Stanford colleagues but did not know Shimony. I nonetheless think of them as a unified trio who jointly inspire me to live up to the examples they set. Columbia's Ernest Nagel (from Chapter 15) passed his passion for intellectual rigor on to his five doctoral protegees. One was Suppes. Another was Isaac Levi, my colleague at Western Reserve, whose strong opinions taught me much, often in vigorous disagreement. A third was Henry Kyburg, at Wayne State during my first faculty position; I had glimpses of his voracious and pyrotechnical intellect and followed some of his work in subsequent years. For being part of that lineage, I am indebted to Nagel too.

I am also often inspired by current and former students. I think of them as mentoring me—informally, to be sure—but sometimes elegantly. Here are a few examples:

A Black student seeking advice told me about a professor of his (no longer at Syracuse):

> I was furious because a racist professor disparaged and embarrassed me in class, but I couldn't think of anything I could do safely. After that I was heading to see a different professor, whose office was a few doors down the hallway from the racist, whose door was ajar. I heard loud talk, so I stopped and listened. It was abuse just like I got. Then the student, a classmate, came out looking really upset: he was a tall, blonde, blue-eyed guy from a prep school on Long Island. So I *didn't* know that prof was racist. Maybe he was, maybe not. What I did know is he's a nasty, abusive bastard who shouldn't be teaching at all. But the main thing I learned was how my own sensitivity led me to conclude what I couldn't defend. Just because

there's a lot of racism, and it affects me every
single day, I can't assume that's what's going on
every time I think I see it.

That student's insight was a valuable reminder of the
importance of being self-critical about our assumptions.
Each of us is in categories that can cause us to think a disappointment is discriminatory because we're in some category
that prompts misogyny, anti-Semitism, xenophobia, or some
other biased hostility. We might be wrong.

At the service desk at Best Buy, my complicated concern
was properly and graciously addressed. Then the service
agent said,

"Professor Gorovitz, I was in your class years
ago. It was the most important class I took."
Surprised, I asked which class; he told me.
Then he added, "You gave me an F. In the first
week you said slackers would not survive. I
was a smug slacker and I always got by before.
That F was the only wake-up call that got
through to me. After that, I worked hard and
I did really well. I have to thank you for that F.
It saved me."

We want to support and encourage all our students.
Sometimes refusing to coddle them is the strongest support.

A student sneezed in class; most classmates reacted by
saying "God bless you" or "Gesundheit." I asked a few students to repeat what they had said and explain why. The
question surprised them; they struggled to answer. Then I
asked what the difference was between the two responses.

They saw that one had theological reference; the other simply wished for good health. Which one they uttered was typically what they heard most often as children. One bilingual student had studied in Poland. I asked what would be said there. She replied in Polish; when I sought translation, she said "Have some vodka!" The students howled with laughter. Then I asked a student from China what classmates would say. She gently replied, "Nothing. Why would we want to call attention to it, and embarrass a student just for sneezing?" This led to a superb discussion about habitual behavior, how well we understand our habits, mindful actions, and Aristotle on the role of habituation as an ingredient of virtue—as well as cultural parochialism.

In a bioethics course, I explored conflicting priorities and values by asking what the students would do with an unexpected gift of a few thousand dollars. One expensively dressed student said, "I'd get my stockbroker's advice." Many students looked aghast. Another, scruffy and earnest, said he'd share it with his extended family to help them meet rent payments. Later, I mentioned people using emergency rooms for primary care because they have no affordable alternative. The student with the stockbroker said, "I never heard of anyone having to use an ER for primary care." The scruffy lad replied, "In my neighborhood I never knew anyone who didn't." These exchanges underscored for me how powerfully students can be one another's teachers and mentors—having far greater influence than had I tried to make the same points.

A startling example of this took place a few blocks away. Bioethics courses should connect the students with clinicians who confront situations like those described in the readings. Sometimes such a guest visits a class, but it's ideal to go to the medical world on a field trip. That's hard with a large class, but mine was small enough to visit the Center for Bioethics and Humanities at Upstate Medical University, a short walk from SU's campus. Our host had read background about each student but wanted a better sense of who they were in person. He asked that each in turn briefly tell something about themselves that might surprise their classmates.

One mentioned a summer job, another a hobby, a third an extra-curricular activity. Then this: "I was kidnaped in Iraq, blindfolded, held captive fifteen days, moved around several times. I did not know if I would live. I kept hearing sounds of weapons. But my family raised enough for the ransom, and I was freed, and we escaped. That is why I am so grateful to be here and in this class." The room was silent, with many students teary. The student up next seemed immobilized. After a long, somber pause, he looked not at the host, but at the Iraqi student, shrugged his shoulders, and said, "Uh . . . I have a dog." The tension in the room resolved, as he continued, "*and*, my dog does tricks!" From that moment, the Iraqi student was not just someone in the class, but a constant reminder to all the others of their comparative privilege and good fortune in having such a courageous and admired classmate.

In each of these unforgettable episodes, the students learned from one another, and I learned as well. More than they know, I remain in their debt.

So, mentoring can be formal or informal, intergenerational, bidirectional, brief or long-lasting. With a shared interest in all aspects of mentoring, my colleagues Joseph Fins, M.D., Cathryn R. Newton, and I co-authored an essay in 2019 with a specific focus on interdisciplinary mentoring, although we acknowledge with gratitude the importance of mentoring within disciplines. Among our concerns is that when mentors are formally assigned to students or junior faculty, the relationship may be more procedural than productive. In part, we said:

> We applaud and advocate mentors who connect ostensibly unrelated disciplines in ways ranging from odd to innovative to visionary. Such pioneers can shape careers by pushing their students to experiment with contrasting disciplines they are then expected to recombine in novel ways . . . Brilliant students often struggle with professional and personal identity. Some of our best students have massive struggles with identity formation. Those students need mentors with unconventional professional identities to help facilitate the intellectual synthesis they seek . . . . Such a mentor must discern the mentee's struggles and perceptions—not so much providing advice as leading the mentee to discovering what is needed to move forward. This is not prescriptively following any well-worn path. It is like going to sea without a nautical chart: not following a protocol but reacting in real time to evolving, unpredictable conditions. Ideal mentors come to know their mentees as individuals and provide scaffolding to hold them up as they develop and sometimes falter. Such mentors can't be assigned; the students must seek and discover them . . . .

We also knew, from our own experiences, that different mentors with different perspectives can open new worlds of understanding:

. . . having multiple mentors with different approaches from different disciplines adds great value to scholars. Contrasting lenses are valuable in classes, too. Co-teaching "LINKED LENSES: Science, Philosophy, and the Pursuit of Knowledge," Gorovitz and Newton engage students in conversations conjoining many disciplines in ways that enrich and alter their understanding of their own disciplines and future prospects. Interdisciplinary mentors can illuminate both the arts and the sciences. For example, the students handle scientific instruments; original letters from figures such as Einstein, Malcolm X, and Tesla; rare original manuscripts by Copernicus and Galileo; and photographs and field notes by Margaret Bourke-White about her legendary images of Gandhi, who required her to learn to weave before agreeing to the photographic studies, and more. Here the metaphor of linked lenses is more than optics. It reflects the magnification of perspective, a benefit in both the sciences and humanities. They also play portions of Leonard Bernstein's CANDIDE in which he discusses the Lisbon earthquake, its connection with Leibniz and Voltaire, and issues of McCarthyism, patriotism, national boundaries, and press freedom. This requires exploring the physics of earthquakes, tsunamis, fire control, and global warming . . .

Our own interdisciplinary mentors re-calibrated our standards of quality and taught us the values of tenacious striving for excellence, of welcoming critical scrutiny, of the essential empowerment of unconventional perspectives that transcend the myopia of a single discipline or field. As Newton recounts:

> MIT strobe pioneer Harold (Doc) Edgerton entered my life when I was 16, a Duke University sophomore. With crated electronics, he arrived in Beaufort, N.C., before our successful search for the long-lost shipwreck of USS *Monitor* off Cape Hatteras. Being assigned to his 4-8 watch (4-8 a.m. and 4-8 p.m.) was transforming. In the long pre-dawn hours, Doc spoke of scientific research and high-speed photography, which he saw as entwined. With an Oscar for film and photographs in the Museum of Modern Art, he thought it obvious: one can be both scientist and world-class artist, and these interactive perspectives enhance each other.

For Fins, also, the integration of scientific and humanistic perspectives fuels creativity for students just as it does for faculty. He reports:

> A pre-med student who loved history worked with me on a bioethics project. Although she was headed toward medicine, history pulled at her heart and mind. She enjoyed the sciences, but broader questions of science in society redirected her aspirations. This became increasingly clear as we worked together on drafts.

She is now completing a graduate degree in the history of medicine, liberated from her more conventional path, I like to think, in part by the interdisciplinarity of what we did together.

The diverse mentoring experiences across our life spans, from youth to later years when we learn from those much younger, flow together like the merging tributaries of a river—constantly adding, as they blend, to our wisdom, creativity, and capacity to impart what we have learned to others. If we have the humility to remember that there's no one from whom we cannot learn, then mentoring and being mentored become inherent to the fabric of our lives. That's the best way to repay what we owe to the early mentors who helped us start toward the successes we have enjoyed.

18

BEAUTIFUL MINDS, MEMORABLE MOVIES, AND ORDINARY OBITUARIES

It does not do to leave a live dragon out of your calcula-
tions, if you live near him.

—*The Hobbit*, J.J.R. Tolkein (1937)

In 2001, Russell Crowe played John Nash in the acclaimed
movie *A Beautiful Mind,* based on a book with the same title
by economic historian Silvia Nasar. Fascinated by the film, I
promptly read the book. Since then, I've encouraged anyone
who's seen the movie to read the book, because it's superb.
But in reading it I saw with surprise that there's little overlap
between the movie, "based on" the book, and the content of
the book. Almost everything in the movie was made up for
the movie. It's not always like that. For example, the gorgeous

2003 film *Girl with a Pearl Earring* about a famous Vermeer painting is not merely "based on" Tracy Chevalier's lovely book of the same name, it is essentially filming, scene by scene, the content of the book.

I loved Nasar's book in part for personal reasons. It's filled with discussions of places I know and even people I knew, including a classmate from MIT who had an important influence on me. As I compared the book and movie, I realized there are three main commonalities: (1) they have the same title, (2) in both, Nash is shown to be a brilliant thinker who won a Nobel Prize, and (3) Nash spends many years in psychiatric hospitals—at times involuntarily—for severe mental illness. That is, because his *mind* was seriously disordered. I was puzzled by my inability to answer this question: If someone had asked me before I had seen the film or read the book to explain the best use of the phrase "a beautiful mind," would I have thought of Nash, who battled a disordered mind for most of his adult life, as the exemplar of that attribute? Did the book and film have the wrong title? I did not know how best to understand the description "a beautiful mind." This haunting puzzlement demanded attention. I created a course titled *Beautiful Minds* to explore that puzzle with a small group of students in our Honors Program.

The students were told:

> We will examine the concept of a beautiful mind, taking that provocative idea from Sylvia Nasar's book of the same title. We will focus on the characteristics of the human mind in general and on the works and lives of a few people with surpassingly powerful intellects. Assignments will include several essays;

regular, active participation in discussions in class is also required. There's much reading, some easy and some quite challenging. You'll love some of the readings and struggle with others and disagree with one another about which readings elicit which response. This course is for students with relentless, wide-ranging curiosity, intellectual tenacity, and a desire to work hard at learning to be both a better thinker and a better writer.

Five paperback books were required (other readings distributed later):

1. *Ex Libris*, by Anne Fadiman
2. *A Beautiful Mind*, by Sylvia Nasar
3. *Surely You're Joking, Mr. Feynman*, by Richard Feynman
4. *Brunelleschi's Dome*, by Ross King
5. *Trace*, by Lauret Savoy

An immediate writing assignment was due in a week:

Write a brief essay in which you address these questions: What are (at least some of) the criteria you would use in deciding that someone has (or had) a beautiful mind? Why did you choose those criteria? What are some criteria you did not choose, but might have? Why did you exclude them? This should be approximately 750-1000 words. Choose each word carefully. Your paper should contain nothing that is not directly responsive to the questions above.

Each student had to propose a research subject whose mind they would assess by whatever criteria they had adopted for considering a mind to be beautiful. That proposal needed my approval, to be sure the choice was possible. (Plato's great-grandmother may have had a beautiful mind, but no presently available resources allow for its assessment.) The proposal also required an initial description of available research resources. The students could modify their criteria and choice of subject along the way; a few did. The initial presentations about their criteria led to vigorous debates; some students thought moral character was central, others thought only intellectual attributes mattered. Some thought impact on the world counted, others thought it irrelevant. Some thought originality of ideas weighed heavily, others thought it didn't matter as long as the ideas arose independently of others. And so on. As these discussions progressed, many students modified their criteria in some respects, but each knew they had sole discretion over what criteria they would use for their projects. Many of the people they chose to investigate were familiar to me. Others I'd not heard of. In every case, I learned an immense amount from the students' interim and final presentations—some of which included finely polished video segments with archival footage of documents, photos, and film clips. The students learned from the presentations within their own semesters; I had the cumulative benefit of all the semesters.

I'm often asked what I teach. People expect a simple answer in familiar terms: American history, organic chemistry, applied statistics, etc. When I say I teach interdisciplinary courses that are not in any specific department or field, they often ask for an example. That's easiest if they've seen the movie about Nash. I inquire; most have seen it, few have read the book, almost none have anything to say about the criteria for judging a mind as beautiful, and nearly all ask about the students' choices of subjects. They were:

Alvin Ailey, Woody Allen, Tadeo Ando, Aristotle, Warren Buffet, George Carlin, Jimmy Carter, Noam Chomsky, Walt Disney, Frederick Douglass, Pope Francis, Viktor Frankl, Sigmund Freud, Theodore Geisel (Dr. Seuss), Malcolm Gladwell, Jane Goodall, Che Guevara, Agnes Gund, Fritz Haber, Anne Hathaway, Jim Henson, Adolph Hitler, Langston Hughes, Steve Jobs, Billy Joel, Frida Kahlo, Helen Keller, Ernst Kirchner, Gary Larson, C.S. Lewis, Warren Littlefield, King Ludwig 2nd of Bavaria, Rene Magritte, Malcolm X, Gabriela Mistral, Jim Morrison, Ryan Murphy, Frederick Nietzsche, Francisco Oller, Pablo Picasso, Sylvia Plath, Shonda Rhimes, Walter Russell, J.D. Salinger, Socrates, Nikola Tesla, Mies van der Rohe, David Foster Wallace, Andy Warhol, Alan Watts, Mike Webster, Louis Zamperini.

One would expect students to conclude that their subjects do qualify for beautiful minds according to the students' criteria. Not always. In a few cases the judgment was negative. That was so with Hitler, chosen because of the effectiveness of his rise to power, his ability to influence vast masses of people, and the magnitude of his impact on history. In this student's analysis, however, no amount of effectiveness could outweigh historically unsurpassed evil. One victim of that evil was Viktor Frankl. As the students read the assigned books, they had to describe the attributes of mind of each of the four authors. The student who chose Frankl as his subject described Frankl as having an attribute from each of the four authors: Feynman was courageous; Brunelleschi was revolutionary; Fadiman was analytical; Nash was brilliant; these four attributes led to a positive assessment of Frankl's mind. This interaction of the readings, student research, and class discussion infused the class with energy and reinforced my contention that everything is related to everything else in substantive and illuminating ways if one does the work to discern or create the relationships.

In a recent iteration of this course, after the students had read all eighteen *Ex Libris* chapters, I asked them each to select one of the sixteen we had not discussed extensively in class and write an analysis of that. Here's the spread:

Sesquipedalians

True Womanhood (3)

Words on a Flyleaf (2)

Nothing New Under the Sun

My Ancestral Castles (2)

Eternal Ink (2)

Sharing the Mayhem

Literary Glutton (2)

Never Do That to a Book

After the students had all read Fadiman's chapter, *Scorn Not the Sonnet*, I explained the structure of a Shakespearean sonnet and the rules defining that form. They each then had to write one—for some the form was familiar and for others it was unknown. Each submitted a sonnet, most abiding by the rules and a few not getting it quite right. I then read them a great sonnet by Elizabeth Barrett Browning (43) and asked whether there might be rules for writing a *great* sonnet. To show that a poem in perfect sonnet form can be dreadful, I wrote this:

I went into the dining hall today

And saw a bunch of stuff I do not like.

I asked if they would take it all away,

And said if not then I would have to strike.

Security then came and hauled me off

And made me pay a big fat ugly fine.

All this because I did not like the trough

Of rotten things on which I will not dine.

Oh! Would some patron saint I've not yet seen,

Take pity and respond to my dire plight

By taking me to find some haute cuisine

To have for dinner almost every night.

Is this too much to hope for, I now ask?

A perfect god would find this a small task.

To my horror, a few students contested my claim that this is poetic junk, I presume because their own gastronomic frustrations distorted their aesthetic judgment. But they all agreed that producing a great sonnet, or judging a sonnet to be great, can no more be done by applying rules than can judging a mind to be beautiful.

In 1991, Albert Brooks starred as Daniel Miller in *Defending Your Life,* which he also wrote and directed. The premise is that after death on Earth, the "little brains" as Earth-dwellers are called, are gathered in Judgment City where an assessment determines whether they are qualified to progress to a higher state of being or should be sent back to Earth (as someone else) for another try. The process of judgment considers a small sample of the person's life—in Daniel Miller's case nine days—the range for other defendants is seven to fifteen days. (Judgment City authorities have video records of every second of the defendant's Earthly life.) One issue raised is what constitutes an adequate sample size; another is how heavily to weigh a sub-sample that may not be representative of the larger whole. The student who chose Jimmy Carter as his subject viewed him as a failed president but noted that one four-year term as president was no longer than an undergraduate's time in college. Asserting that no life or mind should be evaluated solely on the basis of those college years, he assessed Carter's many decades as former president with high praise, leading to a positive judgment.

Defending Your Life earned little at the box office despite moderately favorable reviews. In the thirty years since, it has become increasingly respected, even to the point of being reissued in 2021 in a high definition 4k Blu-ray DVD. In 2016, Brooks told *Rolling Stone,* "I've gotten thousands and thousands of letters of people who had relatives that were dying, or they were dying themselves, and the movie made them feel better. I guess it's because it presents some possibility that doesn't involve clouds and ghostly images."

Judging a mind and judging a life have much in common. Does it matter in assessing a person's mind, work, or life whether its quality or impact were recognized during that person's lifetime? History abounds with examples of assessments that grew or reversed direction over time. The painter Alice Neel (1900–1984) provides a contemporary example; only gradually noticed until late in her life, she is now acclaimed as an artist of unique importance whose works can sell for millions.

The idea of a posthumous review of one's life, with serious consequences, is as old as the mythologies of heaven and hell. It underlies Dante's *Divine Comedy* and appears in contemporary *New Yorker* cartoons. In *Liliom*—the 1909 play by Hungarian Ferenc Molnar, the protagonist is sent back to Earth to right a prior wrong. At least four film versions were made later, but its greatest impact was as the model for the musical *Carousel*, both as a Broadway show and a film. Brooks's Judgment City foreshadows the bardo in George Saunders' *Lincoln in the Bardo*, a pathbreaking book of an entirely new kind that won every award a novel can win.

The idea of post-mortem judges with access to every second of one's life may seem like fanciful fiction but has a chilling edge in this era of social media. Millions now revel in posting images, often videos, of their activities—which often include images of other unwitting participants. Many have come to grief when those images have appeared in ways not anticipated by those who posted them—or because they are in images taken by others who posted them. Even the circumspect are at some risk; the reckless are in serious peril and may have to defend their lives against long odds. In all real lives, the evidence is always mixed if we are able to see more than a misleadingly small sample.

Honest biographies, plays, novels, and movies can give us that mixed evidence in ways that brief snapshot samples never can. Some of those small samples are like eulogies rather than full obituaries, or like indictments based on single events. A recent example is *The Good Boss*, Javier Bardem's ironically titled 2021 film that probes the many interacting threads that weave together a person's character, motivations, actions, self-deception, and reputation—leaving us unable to endorse any uncomplicated judgment of that person.

Many writers, classical to contemporary, have confronted the complexity of assessing a person's mind or character, rejecting simple classifications: there's nothing original in my raising this difficulty. *The Code Breaker: Jennifer Doudna, Gene Editing, and the Future of the Human Race*, by Walter Isaacson (2022), explores this challenge well, as both Doudna and Isaacson wrestle with the nuances of assessing colleagues who have been a mix of friends and enemies, rivals and collaborators. We know we must be tolerant of the imperfections and mistakes of others, yet tolerance has limits, and we must also recognize the intolerable. The Chinese biophysics researcher He Jiankui seemed to be a talented and valuable participant in the CRISPR-Cas 9 research community, even if irrepressibly over-enthusiastic—but later was found to have engaged in unethical and even criminal behavior in his clinical use of gene editing. He was fired, convicted, fined, jailed, and disgraced. Doudna and Isaacson could not judge his accomplishments as outweighing that intolerable failure. (A full account of his downfall appears in MIT's *Technology Review*, December 3, 2019; a more forgiving account of his actions is in *Technology Review*, February 24, 2021.)

I sent the students this message, with the subject line:
   A task you did not plan on but can do now.
   The message read:

> What is going on? This is so odd. I want you to reply to it. Look at it. What do you think this is?

How many words you transmit is up to you. What you say is up to you. Do this by April 24th. Act quickly now if you can.

HINT: irony abounds. You can't fail. Anything you do will comply. What you say is what is right to say.

The students all wrote back, but none (in any semester) has ever discerned what I was doing. In the next class meeting, I asked them to read this passage and say what they think is going on.

Noon rings out. A wasp, making an ominous sound, a sound akin to a klaxon or a tocsin, flits about. Augustus, who has had a bad night, sits up blinking and purblind. Oh what was that word (is his thought) that ran through my brain all night, that idiotic word that, hard as I'd tried to run it down, was always just an inch or two out of my grasp—fowl or foul or vow or voyal?—a word which, by association, brought into play an incongruous mass and magma of nouns, idioms, slogans, and sayings, a confusing, amorphous outpouring which I sought in vain to control or turn off but which wound around my head a whirlwind of a cord, a whiplash of a cord, a cord that would split again and again, would knot again and again, of words without communication or any possibility of combination, words without pronunciation, signification or transcription but out of which, notwithstanding, was brought

forth a flux, a continuous, compact and lucid
flow: an intuition, a vacillating frisson of illu-
mination as if caught in a flash of lightning or
in a mist abruptly rising to unshroud an obvious sign—but a sign, alas, that would last an
instant only to vanish for good.

All sorts of conjectures flowed forth. When I reveal that
the passage is written without the most frequently used letter
of the alphabet—no *e*s here—they are amazed. None of them
noticed that. Then they can understand the irony of the message I had sent them: an e-mail with no *e*. I next assign the task
of sending me a message that follows that constraint; some
sent a few dozen words; some sent a hundred. All reported
it as much harder than they expected, and much more fun.
That passage is a brief excerpt from Georges Perec's novel *A
Void*, a 316-page mystery story written entirely without an *e*.
When I show his book to the class, their amazement soars to
inexpressible astonishment.

This exercise has four benefits:

(1) We all tend to notice what is most easily visible. It can
be equally important to notice what is not there—be it a
Covid antibody, fingerprints on a handgun, or the most
commonly used letter of the alphabet. Our powers of
detection are enhanced if we bear that importance in
mind and actively attend to what might be missing—that
which it will not do to leave out of our calculations; in any
context of decision-making, what's missing can make the
difference between success and failure.

(2) Writing well, especially during the editing stage,
requires seeking and considering alternate ways of

expressing the desired content. Having to write under the "no *e*" constraint helps develop that skill.

(3) Learning about Perec and his work gives the students, none of whom had heard of him, another example of a brilliant and bizarre mind—a new case study to discuss according to their beautiful-mind criteria.

(4) Their own *e*-less responses, and Perec's pyrotechnical imagination, provide a bouquet of creativity that inspires them to think explicitly about how creativity happens and how to expand their own creative capacities.

Here are some examples of what they wrote:

> For communication without that symbol from our talk, why not adopt slang from a distant country?
>
> Arabian: نود مويلا لاوط ةليوط لمج ةباتك يننكمي
> ارارکتو نادأ ةلاسر تقولا مادختساب ايلعف.
>
> Urdu: ا?ک لامعتسا راب ?ئک ں?م ر?ب ر?رحت ?ر?م
> اک ?ا رپ روط ?ںامسج ،سا ،حرط سا روا ?چرگا ،ے? ا?گ
> ے? تالصاوم ?ر?م ر?غب ےئو? ےترک لامعتسا.
>
> ===
>
> Instructor Gorovitz,
>
> An Autumn day
>
> blows my sorrow away.
>
> Soon snow and gray
>
> will cloud my day

and I will pray

for a gay spring ray

===

Wow, look at that! Prof. Gorovitz: a tricky man! That communication was ironic. My communication back to you was not similar, and in fact, a bit silly. Today, I saw a play. This play oddly links to your original communication, for it was a play about communication! In a short summary, it was about a family dynamic in which a child fought against a difficult handicap. It was thought provoking. My family and I had a long talk about it. Boston was simply charming today: sun shining, dogs barking, and dining hall food was NOT in sight.

Tomorrow: back to SU. Looking forward to Monday's class. I am curious in the fun that awaits . . .

===

I was trying to outdo you in this communication, but quickly found out that constructing said communication was much more difficult than I had thought it would. My ivory flag is rising as I think, good morrow.

===

Hi, This is a fun but difficult task. It is hard to think of words for this communication. But wait, I did accomplish what I was told to do with this communication anyways. Yay, not as hard as I thought!

===

I don't know what to think. I'm so lost and without words. I don't know what to say. I couldn't say anything that could in any way show how lost I truly am. I know that you will know just as much confusion as I, with having this odd communication in your inbox.

===

What's up? This communication is hard. I don't know how to form a long communication in this way. I will try though. I am curious about what is going on on Friday. What will our class do? What food is it? Hmmm. This is difficult. This also is bad writing. I am sorry about that. It is hard to form a communication. I now know why this is ironic.

===

Thanksgiving is drawing nigh! I await in anticipation in joining my family and companions again. My mind drifts off to thoughts of food, fun and laughs. Aroma of gravy and corn which I miss most! For now I must turn back to the world of motion in physics.

I had also asked the students to identify the most salient attributes of Anne Fadiman's mind, based solely on the content of *Ex Libris*. I then had them write a comparable description of their own attributes of mind. For each such attribute, I asked whether they wanted to enhance, diminish, or modify that attribute. Or preserve that attribute as it is. Finally, they realized that all along my secret quarry was not for them to understand the concept of a beautiful mind, but to encourage them to be thoughtful, reflective, and imaginative about their own minds, the choices that await them, and the lives they will lead.

In a different course, I asked the students to bring an obituary to the next class. They had questions about why and how, all of which I declined to answer. I simply reiterated: bring an obituary. At that next class, most had obits clipped or copied from newspapers. I asked one to read his aloud, then asked if anyone had a younger or older death to report. The range was from infants to centenarians. We considered the kinds of lives described; some were people of renown, others ordinary folks with no public presence. The students were interested in these findings but still puzzled about why we were doing it. Their next assignment explained that.

Emphasizing that the stories of our lives are shaped partly by the choices we make and partly by external factors beyond our control, I asked them to imagine the lives awaiting them. Each student was then to write her or his own one-page obituary in three versions, one reflecting their loftiest hopes, another reflecting what they saw as most probable, a third reflecting their darkest fears. Two responses remain most vivid for me. For one guy, all three versions described returning to his hometown in New Jersey with employment in a local company. His most likely outcome was a life in middle management there, but his hope was for upper management and his fear was lower middle management. That disheartening, tedious, gloomy outlook was in sharpest contrast with the response of a woman whose aspirational outcome was to become a distinguished lawyer, political activist, and philanthropist—rising to the US Senate and ultimately to the Supreme Court. Her worst outcome was to be admitted to her first-choice law school and in the summer before matriculating there being killed by a drunken driver.

With the help of Ann Marshall, then a doctoral student in the Social Sciences program and now a research librarian at Purdue, Fort Wayne, we analyzed 156 of the obituaries. Some results were unsurprising. Ideal lives ended with gentle deaths, serene endings to fulfilling lives. Feared lives often ended in troubling or tragic ways. Some feared lives were brief; others, devoid of purpose or enjoyment, seemed to drag on endlessly. Ideal lives were described with richness of detail; expected lives were not and lacked the drama of the best and worst outcomes. Images of grandeur, power, wealth, and acclaim pervade the ideal lives, reflecting the values of the larger culture. Given the charge to think big, many students imagined themselves as successful corporate or political figures, stars in the NBA or NFL, or famous poets, authors, actors or models. In those lives, one does not just go to the Olympics, but "wins the gold by an amazing margin." Almost without exception, the students envisioned them-selves sharing their success with others. Forty-four described themselves as married; all but four mentioned children. In these ideal narratives, difficult choices were unnecessary. Challenges were gracefully overcome without struggle or hardship. Even death, which comes peacefully in their sleep, or in the garden in the arms of a loved one, or "shortly after learning that the donor heart she declined has saved a young boy's life." In contrast, death in the feared lives looms large and ominous. Students wrote of prolonged disease, painful ailments, automobile accidents, drowning, cancer, murders.

One dies at nineteen "with asthma, gasping for air in her dormitory room." Many fail to finish college, and without a degree have lives of tedious disappointment. Few of these stories consider that choices were made poorly. Mostly, the disappointing outcomes were attributed to external factors; the odds were stacked against them, and their lives were out of their control and beyond their influence.

In the expected life obituaries, almost all students seemed satisfied with the lives they anticipate and describe lives rich with family, creativity, and career in which they are well-respected by friends and neighbors. Their expectations are essentially optimistic. (I suspect that would be less likely now, given the impact of the Covid pandemic.) Only eight students described hardship or sacrifice in the expected lives, which resembled the ideal lives much more closely than the feared lives. In many cases, the outcomes were milder versions of the ideal, such as one who hopes to be a national TV news anchor but expects to be a local broadcaster. Some students came from highly educated and affluent backgrounds; others were from disadvantaged backgrounds of various kinds, including being first in the family to go beyond high school. We found no correlation between the backgrounds and how lofty their aspirations were. For a few, the best and worst lives were close to their expectations. For others, with a much richer imagination about possibilities, the range was immense.

Many students found the assignment difficult and even disturbing. Most reported discussing it with friends, roommates, and sometimes family, as well as classmates. They also seemed keenly interested in what we found in their obituaries. This provided an effective basis for discussing the extent to which, and the ways in which, the lives we lead are amenable to influence by the choices we make. Students are typically naive about factors such as luck, chance, control, responsibility, uncertainty, self-deception, and regret. They often think, wrongly, that difficult decisions must be important and important decisions must be difficult. They also think the quality of a decision can be inferred from its outcome, and that good things that happen to them are their accomplishments, but bad things are inflicted by circumstance. Their willingness to explore such issues flowed from having them imagine and write about the range of possible lives ahead.

As we think about our minds—what they are like, what we would like them to be—our sense of the future is influenced by how expansively we can imagine the range of possibilities. It's the same with the lives we will lead, whether we are contemplating the future at eighteen or at eighty. The future we pursue must be one we can envision, so the more creatively we can envision future lives and assess their appeal, the more likely we will judge our minds and our lives to have been beautiful, as the time for those obituaries approaches.

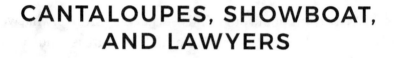

19

CANTALOUPES, SHOWBOAT, AND LAWYERS

Tote that barge, lift that bale, get a little drunk and you land in jail.

—Jerome Kern and Oscar Hammerstein,
Showboat (1927)

At the California State University at Northridge, where I had been invited to speak in October 2002, I met a high school student who had recently finished a summer program for talented young writers, led by a professor they adored. The fifteen students in that highly selective program had one final assignment, to submit an essay on a topic of their choice. Although they would not be together after handing in those essays, they secretly agreed that whatever their topics, each would use the word "cantaloupe" once. They conjectured mirthfully about how many essays the professor would read before realizing that something was up. I admired their creativity, humor, and ability to delight in imagining a result they would never see. Caring about an unseen future is common in older people when they write wills, plan bequests, establish endowments, or even relinquish children in searing refugee situations in the confident hope that those children will have better life prospects. It's less common among teenagers, who are more prone to care only about the very short-term future. I was impressed by the unusual maturity of these thoughtful youngsters.

This was not the first time in California that thinking about cantaloupes prompted me to reflect on serious matters. One classmate in my first year of graduate school was raised in Arizona, the son of a fundamentalist Baptist minister, within a culture that prohibited such moral errors as drinking, dancing, going to movies, and questioning authority. (I'll call him AZ.) An imposing figure, tall, broad-shouldered and powerful, he exuded an aura of physical strength and mental intensity. Starting at sixteen years, he had worked long, hard hours in the cantaloup industry loading heavy wooden crates of cantaloups into railroad freight cars and long-haul trucks that would take the produce to markets. By the time he entered college, he had started to consider the possibility that the authorities who had guided and constrained his choices might be flawed. Still in their grip, he arrived at Westmont College—a high quality liberal arts college which embraced the fundamentalist thought that infused his earlier education. But Westmont was in California and that made all the difference. The college was accredited, which required that all students take a course in California history. For a student as intellectually powerful as AZ, the course was shallow and narrow. Yet it yielded one important moment. An exam given by a temporary professor contained this question:

> Prior to the Gold Rush in 1849, the population
> of California was less than _____

AZ answered 10^{10}. The professor had lifted a paragraph from the textbook and left blanks to be filled in by the students. (He had not said "According to our textbook . . .") AZ saw instantly that if any answer was correct, as a point of logic his had to be, but was marked wrong. He went to the professor, expecting to have a few points restored, pointing out that the population of California was larger than in 1849, and yet much less than 10^{10}. The professor dismissed AZ's claim saying AZ should not challenge his authority. This episode was just one small part of the erosion of AZ's beliefs, but important enough for him to tell me about it years later. After college, he returned to Arizona and earned a master's degree at the University of Arizona. At Stanford, his struggles with identity and belief continued, leading to divorce, remarriage, and an extensive transformation of lifestyle. But his strength of intellect and character were unchanged. Of the eighteen students in our entering doctoral class, he was among the five who completed the program; he then had a fine career as a professor and department chair. For sixty years I have admired his intellectual and moral courage as an example of pursuing the best available evidence and following it wherever it leads, however discomforting that journey may be. (I've also seen too many people who reminded me of that history teacher, about whom I know nothing more than that one story AZ told.)

Loading bales of cotton onto a boat under severe constraints isn't so different from loading crates of cantaloupes onto a train under severe constraints. In one case, getting a little drunk would land one in jail; in the other, getting a little drunk would prompt clerical and possibly divine punishment landing one in a place worse than jail. The song "Ol' Man River" was written for Paul Robeson, who sang it in 1928 to worldwide acclaim in the London premier of *Showboat*. In a meeting of the Linked Lenses class described above, we asked how many students knew who Paul Robeson was. None did, although the class was diverse and included an African American student. We explained that Robeson was an All-American football star, later an NFL professional and a graduate of Columbia Law School who completed his law degree while playing professional football. But he quickly left the practice of law because of the racism he encountered, and his solidarity with disadvantaged populations led him to adopt increasingly critical views of American society. The US government suspended his passport while he was abroad, and for many years he was unable to return to this country. He was erased from American history.

When we explained this to the class, one student was trembling with anger. A white male from a prestigious public school on Long Island, he said:

> Robeson is IMPORTANT! His story is IMPORTANT! It's part of American history. How can it be that I never heard of him? That's not acceptable. And what really *really* upsets me is that if I never heard of him, what else that's important don't I know about, that I don't even know I don't know about?

After Robeson was denied access to this country, he performed in Canada at the Peace Arch border crossing in British Columbia. Tens of thousands of American fans massed on the American side to hear the concert, and artistic creativity and appreciation prevailed over political paranoia. That

Showboat itself misrepresents the circumstances of enslaved people and thus contributes to a narrative that falsifies history is also an ironic and important part of the story.

François-Marie Arouet, using the *nom de plume* Voltaire, wrote the scathing anti-establishment satire *Candide* (1759). Leonard Bernstein, as composer, with Lillian Hellman as principal librettist, transformed it into a Broadway musical (1956). Voltaire and Bernstein also had their passports suspended for making government powers uncomfortable. When our students heard all this, they understood the generality and contemporary relevance of the Robeson story. We played a CD of Robeson singing *Ol' Man River*, and many in the class were visibly moved. Although Robeson died in 1965, once one hears that distinctive voice it endures in one's mind, and his sound, like his story, lives on. This led to an eerie, otherworldly experience. Our head of libraries invited friends to a garden party; by the time I arrived, many guests were there, with others still to come. As I walked across the garden, I suddenly heard Paul Robeson speaking just a few steps behind me. It wasn't Robeson, of course, but his son, Paul Robeson Jr., who sounded just like his father and was related by marriage to the librarian.

That acoustical confusion was a familiar phenomenon. When I was in high school, it was said that, on the phone, my father—(like Robeson, a lawyer)—and I sounded the same. One day I answered a call, and after a pause his client—(an observant Catholic)—asked, "Is this the father or the son?" I replied, "They're both busy. It's the Holy Ghost. May I take a message?" I wasn't sent to jail or the inferno, but I was gently advised that my answering skills needed improvement.

Almost all my father's professional life was in Boston. However, during the Second World War, he was Chief Counsel to the Leather, Fur and Fibers Branch and the Wool Section of the Office of Price Administration in Washington, D.C. An industry lobbyist came to recommend a specific pricing decision and said, "That paper bag I put on your desk contains $25,000. If you can assure me that you'll follow our recommendation, I can forget to take the bag when I leave." Seconds later the lobbyist and his bag were thrown out of the office, and a bit of family lore was created. Spiro Agnew's eagerness to accept such bags conjured a very different scene. (When I told this story in class once, a student said, "I'm from Staten Island. My parents' friends were delivering those bags.")

My father was an immigrant from eastern Europe, and the FBI's background check for his pending government appointment was extensive. My request in the 1990s for his file under the Freedom of Information Act yielded dozens of pages, most of which were almost entirely redacted. Government fear of possibly dissenting citizens is persistent across time and space—one reason why strong, independent, investigative journalism is essential. It is always under threat. Indeed, Vladimir Putin's first assignment as a new KGB agent was to suppress dissent—a tactic to which he has remained ruthlessly committed.

Before social media fractured us into separated informational tribes, the three major television networks competed for the same vast national population of viewers. A producer for one of the morning programs (I think it was ABC's *Good Morning America*)—called to ask whether I would be willing to appear on their program. I agreed, and was then asked what position I would take on the topic in question (whatever that was). I explained my views, and the producer said she would get back to me. The next day she reported that I would not be chosen for the program because my views were too reasonable. They wanted participants with extreme views so there would be sharper conflict to hold the viewers' attention.

I expressed appreciation for her candor, but not for the insight this exchange gave me into the values behind this masquerade of providing quality broadcast journalism.

Our student didn't know about Robeson because the sanitized version of American history he was taught excluded that information. His ignorance wasn't his fault. Some ignorance, however, is culpable. If a physician mishandles a case in ignorance of recently published relevant information, that violates a responsibility to be aware of current best practices. The same applies to university athletic directors who try to evade responsibility for sexual harassment by claiming they were unaware of problems or complaints at lower levels of the organization; they had relied on trusted staff who let them down. These evasive efforts properly fail because the directors have an affirmative responsibility to know of such matters.

We are all ignorant of most of what is known; that's why we turn to authorities we trust, such as experts, websites, or printed material. Sometimes our ignorance is easily correctable: If I don't know the weather forecast, I can check it, learn that rain is ahead, and take my umbrella. Or if I don't know whether my patient has a specific allergy, I can get a DNA analysis and learn that the standard drug is too risky but an alternate seems fine. But tracking the path of ignorance isn't any easier than tracking the path of a hurricane. In our course, when reviewing the devastation of hurricane Katrina, we asked: What was known as the storm approached? What was not known but could have been known? What was it culpable not to have known? We asked who should bear what responsibility for their own culpable ignorance or for the avoidable ignorance of others, and who is trying to blame others for their own failings, as people in power so often do.

Such questions reveal the need to explore strategies for not overlooking what is dangerous to miss—more dangerous than the absence of an *e*. We need to unearth what people in positions of power don't want us to know, while recognizing that confidentiality is often justified. In any situation, most of what we don't know is not relevant to our concerns. So we must have good selective judgment about what additional knowledge to seek. No physician, faced with a complicated choice, would call for all available medical tests to be done. She needs to order those that can shed light on this specific case, being careful not to overlook those that are not typically thought relevant to such cases yet in rare situations could be. It's similarly reasonable for an undecided diner to ask a server whether anything on the menu is unavailable; it is not relevant to ask the ages of the chef's children, if any. Yet even our judgment about what further information is relevant may reflect biases or be based on unjustified assumptions. The differential treatment and testing decisions about women with long-Covid symptoms, depending on whether they are white or women of color, exemplifies such bias. That's where our strategies come into play.

In a course on decision-making, I gave the two dozen students this problem:

> You must cross a body of flowing water of unknown depth and current speed, two lanes wide, to meet a commitment on the other side. Write down all the ways you can think of to do that.

(Reader: You can try this now. Before reading on, set this book aside and jot down the first half-dozen ideas that occur to you. If you are as adventurous as I suspect you are, you'll find this useful.)

I then asked the students each to report on any one of their ideas. These included the obvious: swim across, find a rowboat, build a raft, rent a helicopter—and the less obvious: tunnel under the water, arrange for parasailing, bounce across from a large trampoline. When they had spoken, I asked the whole class how many had heard another student mention an idea that hadn't occurred to them. Every student raised a hand. I proposed finding a circus that can make you the person shot from a cannon and asked whether anyone had thought of that. No one had. In a later year, the course had 134 students. I could only sample a small subset of their ideas, but the results were the same; they all heard ideas from others they had not thought of themselves.

One clear message is that our awareness of what's possible in a decisional situation can be expanded greatly by hearing from others who think about it differently. That fuels the familiar medical practice of getting a second opinion, which often redirects thinking and has saved many lives. The value of alternate opinions in medical decisions is unmistakable. Its broader value is often overlooked. One simple example: an international student, completing her Ph.D., applied for jobs with strong support from her doctoral advisor. She accepted an offer in this country and the employer enthusiastically began planning for her arrival. Shortly before she was to begin work, she was astonished to receive an offer from her home country for what was the job of her dreams in every respect. She knew that it would not come her way again. She saw two options: (1) decline the new offer on the grounds that she was already committed to a job, and then begin her career not with enthusiasm but an ongoing sense of loss and grieving, or (2) take the new offer, backing out of her commitment, betraying her advisor, and perhaps damaging that advisor's credibility for the future, thus going home not with unalloyed joy but with a burden of guilt and self-recrimination. She was afraid that even discussing this with her advisor would do irreparable damage.

She sought my advice. I said she was asking the wrong person, and suggested she tell the person who had already hired her that she would honor her commitment but wanted to convey this new information to explain what might seem to be dampened enthusiasm. She had not thought of this and agreed to try it. The new employer readily said, approximately, "It's wonderful news for you. Of course, you should accept that offer. It's a bit inconvenient for us, but greatly important for you. We're disappointed not to have you, but we'll soon find another excellent candidate who can join us without reservations." That's what happened; it took only an outside perspective pointing out a previously unseen possibility.

A second message can be especially hard for talented students to accept: generating wild, impractical, unrealistic ideas is not a mistake, but a liberating catalyst for creativity. *Evaluating* ideas—one's own or others—is different from *generating* ideas and shouldn't inhibit the consideration of ideas that may seem bonkers. Sometimes those ideas yield the most important successes. The history of science recounts many examples of oddball conjectures—often by under-valued women such as Nobel Laureate Barbara McClintock, Rachel Carson, and Marie Tharp—later validated as para-digm-changing contributions to scientific progress.

Seeing anew from unfamiliar perspectives is impeded when those perspectives are suppressed, as in the historical narratives that omit Paul Robeson, the role of women writers and scientists, or the complicity of university founders in the slave trade. Government officials, politicians, and corpo-rate executives go to great lengths and expenditure—(often hiring lawyers and public relations consultants)—to obfuscate, deflect, and mislead when their interests would be undermined if an accurate perspective came to light. Public interest lawyers, often pro bono, strive to reveal the facts through such measures as Freedom of Information inquiries and discovery processes. But independent investigative journalism is the most essential antidote to such suppression of diverse perspectives. That's why autocratic leadership views a free press as an enemy of the people, and contrives to control, disparage, and influence it. Independent journalism is an endangered species in the ecology of information, yet it is a keystone species—one on which the health of the rest of the system depends in interconnected ways. It must be defended vigorously, as Rachel Maddow's dazzling podcast series *Ultra* (2022) has demonstrated with unsurpassed force.

It need not be the *New York Times*; independent student journalism has often been the force that led to important disclosures and constructive change. Long ago, at Syracuse University, two student journalists wrote an exposé about our then chancellor, who, although admirable in many ways, was volatile, hypersensitive, and vindictive. She did not have the hide of an elephant, nor even the skin of a cantaloupe. Whatever the show, she needed to be the unchallenged star. She excoriated those two students publicly, accused them of unethical behavior, and required her cowering deans to endorse a statement defending her against the students' claims. But their award-winning article won national acclaim and launched their careers as successful journalists. Even the chancellor's staff-writers and lawyers could not keep the curtain from coming down on the false narrative that she was open-minded, reasonable, and fair. Brava to those student journalists, and to independent investigative journalists everywhere.

HOME PLATE, THE CHEESE LADY, AND, AGAIN, BAD SONNETS

Little things mean a lot.

—Kitty Kallen (1954)

The uses and limits of regulations and rules have interested me since my student days. As a sophomore in a fraternity, I experienced this: the freshmen, only the freshmen, were required to wear a tie and jacket at dinner. Their sense of injustice was matched by their intrepid protest. They posted guards at the doors and windows, complied strictly with the regulations, and showed up wearing ties and jackets. Just ties and jackets. Nothing else. Picture that.

When the division manager at Lockheed Aircraft (See Chapter 8) said I did not have a high enough level of security clearance to see the report I had written, he was following regulations; I could not get it back.

Of course, he wasn't French. A few decades ago, when I was often in Geneva, I worked with Bill Lowrance—a discerning, insightful, and bemused American colleague. His office was in Geneva and his apartment a short walk away, across the border in France. He described their differing cultural attitudes toward rules, regulations, and laws by saying the Swiss stop at stop signs, look both ways before crossing, park only as allowed, and understand the train schedule to describe reality, whereas the French consider rules, regulations, schedules, and laws to be interesting suggestions.

In graduate school I wondered what it is about regulations that seems so often to be a barrier to any semblance of common sense. I started then to think about barriers, as well as rules and regulations. As an academic administrator, I often focused as much on removing barriers to constructive action as on providing incentives, realizing that what faculty often need leaders to do is just get the bureaucratic obstructions out of their way so they can get on with doing the good work they are dedicated to doing. Of course, some kinds of barriers, such as barrier islands, can just disappear naturally. I'll return to that shortly.

I had the privilege of presenting a keynote address at a PRIMR meeting in Boston (Public Responsibility in Medicine and Research) in the shadow of Fenway Park, a sacred place since my youth. On that occasion, the title of my remarks was "Senator Proxmire, the Baltimore Orioles, and the National Research Agenda." William Proxmire, a Democratic Senator from Wisconsin, issued monthly "Golden Fleece" awards to projects he viewed as wasting government resources—168 in all. Reacting to his often worthy but sometimes wacky choices, I cited the Orioles to make a point about algorithmic decision-making and the fallibility of predictive judgment. I said, approximately:

Senator Proxmire, in his "Golden Fleece Awards" comments, suggested that, if the National Science Foundation had its act together, it would support just those research projects that led to constructive results—the ones that worked. After all, what are they being paid for? That leads me to the Baltimore Orioles. When that debate about the selection of scientific research was taking place, I called the Orioles. I said, "You have the best farm team system in professional baseball. I want to know how successful you are in signing new hires. I know that for someone to get a contract in the Orioles' system and become professional, it is not nearly enough just to be the best ball player a high school has ever produced, or to be an all-state star. It is not enough just to be fabulously good. You have to be immensely better than that to become professional." They said, "That's right, and some years are much better than others. In a bad year everybody falls by the wayside." I asked, "How many, out of a hundred signed, on average, ultimately will wear the Orioles uniform and play in the major leagues?" The reply was, "Well, the range is about one to two percent." I was tempted to ask, "Isn't that inept? Why don't you just give contracts to the ones who are going to make it?" Of course, everyone understands why that is impossible and knows that they have to take risks because good predictive ability about such outcomes does not and cannot exist. Even people who are deeply stupid about how science works seem to understand the baseball analogy, and can make the transfer—at least, if they are led to it. The general point is about uncertainty and the taking of risks.

I will continue the baseball theme, starting—as one ought—at home plate. In describing Chief Justice John Roberts shortly after his confirmation, the eminent *New York Times* reporter Linda Greenhouse wrote, "That raises the question of whether the chief justice's performance conforms to his own stated goal: to be a 'minimalist' judge who decides no more than necessary, an umpire simply calling balls and strikes." My late colleague David Potter at that time had thirty-five years of experience as an umpire—experience which served him well as our associate dean for Student Services. He took exception to that account of umpiring. In response to Linda Greenhouse, he wrote:

> While it is true that there is a detailed rule book and several case books, much of what an umpire decides is based on circumstances, interpretation, unwritten "common law" which one learns on the field. In many respects the situation is like that of the beat cop. Were he or she simply to enforce all the laws as written, the officer wouldn't last a month, and shouldn't. Both the umpire and the officer on the street have a much more basic and important task than strictly enforcing the law: They must each help assure that the community in one case, and the ballfield in the other, are able to function as intended.

The thrust of Potter's observation wasn't that rules and regulations are unimportant or to be scorned, but that they are only a part of the story—tools to use in pursuit of larger objectives with underlying values. Strict compliance with those tools can undermine those objectives. A similar point is made by Nobel Laureate Amartya Sen in his 2022 memoir, *Home in the World*. He cites the fourth century Sanskrit classic play *Mricchakatika*, by Shudraka, which explains justice thus:

> The distinction is between the concepts of justice represented respectively by two Sanskrit terms: *niti* and *nyaya*. Among the principal uses of *niti* are the virtues of following well-defined rules and organizational propriety. In contrast with *niti*, the term *nyaya* stands for a comprehensive concept of realized justice. In that view, the roles of institutions, rules and organizations, important as they are, have to be assessed in a broader and more inclusive perspective on the world that actually emerges from the process of justice, not just the institutions or rules we happen to have.

The limitations of rules and regulation, about baseball or justice, are special cases of a larger category: the limitations of algorithmic analysis generally—of rule-based, quantitative assessment of matters that may instead require the kind of approach that Potter advocates.

Now, the cheese lady. This is no allusion to Monty Python, although it could be. Long ago, I visited my friend Marty Gellert in the lab he directs at the National Institutes of Health. (At ninety-four, he still directs that lab and continues to publish important work.) He put a piece of paper on the counter and, handing me a well-sharpened pencil, asked me to sign my name without touching the paper with my hands or dotting the *i*. I did. He then picked that paper up with tweezers and weighed it on a laboratory scale. We looked at the digital readout, which had many numbers. He put the paper back on the counter, and said, "Now, again without touching the paper with your hands, dot the *i*." I dotted the *i*. We weighed the paper again, did the subtraction, and determined the weight of the dot of the *i*. For molecular genetics, that degree of precision—that little thing—matters.

A few months later, at the cheese counter in an Amish shop, I said, "I'd like half a pound of that cheddar, please." A straight-faced Amish woman took a lovely instrument with a curved blade and a wooden handle on each side, approached a large block of cheese and pondered it carefully, and then cut off a segment. She put it on a scale, which read .50. Astonished, I said, "You've done this before. I want to see it again. So, I'd like half a pound of the Swiss cheese, also." Deadpan, she cut the Swiss cheese, weighed it on the scale, and saw .46. And she looked me straight in the eyes and monotonically said, "It's the holes."

Suppose instead she had said, "Sorry, I'll do it again," got .53, and then said, "Let me just trim that a little," got another .50—only to say, "It still might be a little over, but below the detection limits of my scale. I'd better get one of those scales from NIH." Such passion for precision would be pure pathology. This would be someone in the wrong line of work, on the brink of not being in that line of work anymore. Such a little difference doesn't matter. It's a marginal difference that means nothing. However, if we go to a neurosurgeon because of a growing pressure on the brain, we do not want to hear, "Well, that's close enough, anyway." An extremely small difference in cranial pressure, as that pressure approaches the limits of elasticity, can make all the difference that matters between success and failure, between life and death. We need good judgment to understand how much a little difference will matter in deciding what level of precision a context demands.

A sophisticated understanding of precision is not about maximizing accuracy in all contexts. It's about the relationship between little things and big things. It's about the impact of small differences at the margins and it demands a kind of experienced judgment for which there are no algorithms. Without that judgment, there's little chance of making the distinction well between doing a task flawlessly and doing it unacceptably, whether the task is selling cheese, umpiring a baseball game, or doing surgery. There's no more chance than a computer has of being an inspired poet, writing a sonnet of enduring beauty and power. The new developments in AI-generated writing are impressive and intriguing, but still fall far short of matching the magic of a literary master.

Indeed, that difference between merely doing a task in compliance with the rules and doing it well is nowhere better illustrated than by the example of crafting a sonnet, discussed earlier (Chapter 18). Imagine a government Office for Protection from Bad Sonnets. The regulators from that office would check to see if the rules had been followed— what else could they do? At universities throughout the country, at least those whose faculty write or teach sonnets with support from federal funds, there would be concern to be in compliance with the regulations. Some examples will help, but let's start with the regulations.

A sonnet is a fourteen-line poem, typically of either the Italian (that is, Petrarchan) or English (that is, Shakespearean) form, defined by distinct rules. The Italian form is divided into the octave and the sestet, each with a specific rhyme scheme. The English sonnet—which we consider here—has three quatrains and a couplet, with the typical rhyme-scheme being:

abab cdcd efef gg.

The last two lines, often epigrammatic, reflect on the content of the first twelve.

There's no better example of the Shakespearian sonnet, of course, than one by Shakespeare. Here's #55, called "Not marble nor the gilded monuments":

> Not marble, nor the gilded monuments
> Of princes, shall outlive this powerful rhyme;
> But you shall shine more bright in these
>   contents
> Than unswept stone, besmear'd with sluttish
>   time.
> When wasteful war shall statues overturn,
> And broils root out the work of masonry,
> Nor Mars his sword, nor war's quick fire shall
>   burn
> The living record of your memory.
> 'Gainst death, and all oblivious enmity
> Shall you pace forth; your praise shall still
>   find room
> Even in the eyes of all posterity
> That wear this world out to the ending doom.
> So, till the judgment that yourself arise,
> You live in this, and dwell in lovers' eyes.

That, I submit, is as vividly clear an example of a fine sonnet as one can find. In starkest contrast is the sonnet I wrote about the dining hall. I did not exactly write it to illuminate Hume's discussion of the problem of evil in his *Dialogues Concerning Natural Religion,* but to mark the contrast between a sonnet that merely complies with the regulations, and one that is any good. My dreadful sonnet complies strictly with the rules and would pass muster with our new Office of Protection from Bad Sonnets. Some serious suffering would result from that approval. But that is not the worst problem here. Let's revisit that authentically fine sonnet, #55. Imagine this complaint from an angry stickler to the member of Congress from his district, thus:

> Dear Congressman Thwartlots:
>
> What is going on with your Office of Protection from Bad Sonnets? I am trying to uphold standards we can all be proud of. I represent the Center for Sonnetarian Integrity, and we vote. And I see that in Shakespeare's sonnet #55, there is a problem that your overpaid bureaucrats have just missed, or don't care about, and I don't even know which is worse. Look at these lines yourself:
>
> Not marble, nor the gilded monuments
> Of princes, shall outlive this powerful rhyme;
>
> The first line has ten syllables. Does the second? You're in Congress, for Heaven's sake. You ought to know something about power. Can you count? Try saying "power" in one syllable. You can't. That line has eleven syllables, and this sonnet, I don't care who wrote it, is no example to hold up for our young people today, who have to learn the difference between what follows the rules and what does not . . . ."

I'll spare you the rest of this very long letter, but not the rest of the story. Congressman Thwartlots makes a call or two, and OPBS rescinds approval of sonnet 55. One university, teaching that sonnet with the support of a federal grant, hangs tough and insists it is a good sonnet. Thwartlots (from Florida) tweets a complaint that this university is guilty of being woke. OPBS initiates an inquiry. The provost's office gets involved, committees form, hearings ensue, and now various people— some of them well-educated, some of them elected officials, and a few of them even both—are spending time assessing and disputing various pronunciations of "power"—while they are really thinking about the press, the risk-managers, and the flow of cash. Local Sonnet Monitoring Committee members resign, and others refuse to serve, because they have come to see such committee work as futile or even dangerous. That is even more damaging than having to hear my fully compliant, technically perfect, really bad sonnet.

One dose of sensible critical judgment would have avoided these problems. But that's only possible when a system of oversight allows for good judgment. If there is no place for judgment, even a minor deviation from regulations can lead to serious storms of accusations, recriminations, distractions, and unproductive interventions. Serious storms do serious damage.

One serious storm, Hurricane Katrina, was unexpected in its specificity yet of a kind that was expected and even predicted. Among its consequences has been a flood of analysis, including a focus on some ostensible non-compliance with medical regulations in its immediate aftermath. Steven Miles, among the nation's most thoughtful, humane, and eloquent physicians, provided this perspective:

> When disaster and medical ethics collide, when
> the respirators, the labs, the x-rays go dark, the

serum does not arrive, the extra sitting nurses disappear, the telecommunications turn off, the on-line medical records become as unobtainable as the paper files in the flooded basement, the medical ethics landscape is changed—not in a way that suspends the ethical rules of practice but in ways that can make them impossible to logically use.

This is not a screed against respect for regulations, but against regulations blindly invoked in contexts of disaster, like the immediate aftermath of Katrina, the worst days of the Covid pandemic, and the current horrors in Ukraine, Turkey, Syria, and too many other places. Once in a while, unpredictably, there will be disasters, future Katrinas, tsunamis, earthquakes, and plagues. When they occur, there may or may not be villains, and non-compliance with regulations may or may not be part of the story. It makes no sense to ask only whether regulations were followed, without making the crucially important, and sometimes subtle, distinctions among the various ways non-compliance can occur.

Wrestling with such stressful matters can prompt one to want to lock the office, turn off the cell phone, and just head for the beach. But that's not always possible. One of the harms caused by Katrina was the complete disappearance of some small islands in the Gulf of Mexico, plus extensive damage to many beaches. That's distressing because we care about beaches, for many reasons. We love them, yet know that they are dynamic, ever-changing, often fragile interfaces between land and sea. Let's consider going to the beach on one of the beautiful barrier islands off the coast of North Carolina. You buy some expensive beachfront property there and build a fine house safely behind the high tide margin. Time passes, there's a storm once in a while, a lot of sand washes away, and one day your house is no longer on the dry side of the water's edge. It is largely *in* the water even at low tide and starts breaking apart. That sort of thing happens, increasingly often. Perhaps you had said, "Hey! My beach is eroding. Call the Corps of Engineers. Build a seawall. Nourish the beach with trucks of sand. Protect my private property and do it with taxpayer subsidy." This also happens often. And sometimes, the whole island just goes away, as when Katrina was raging.

The leading expert on beachfront erosion is Orrin Pilkey of Duke University. He and Linda Pilkey-Jarvis wrote a splendid book, with the captivating title *Useless Arithmetic* (2007). Pilkey is an accomplished scientist, so this is intriguing. The main theme is that there is a widespread and dangerous attraction to false claims of precision and accuracy, and that mathematical models in particular, although much revered, are not adequate for predicting Earth surface changes. The authors offer as a stunning case study the example of Bruun's Rule for calculating expected shoreline erosion. It is based on provably bad assumptions and leads to embarrassing consequences, yet it has been adopted throughout the world as a tool for planning. The reasons for its mystifying and indefensible adoption, they point out, are that it is available, is simple to apply, has no serious competitors, and has at least a thin veneer of ostensible precision. That is apparently enough.

It's not that the Pilkeys want us to abandon empiricism or make guesses uninformed by evidence. Instead, they want informed qualitative judgment. We can, based on evidence, justify claims about trends, directions, and proportionality. And we can do that best if we have some reasonable judgment about what makes good sense—rather than following a formulaic approach applied algorithmically but detached from reality—especially when that formula is made sufficiently malleable—by using fudge factors—to accommodate any observable data. That makes it essentially unfalsifiable. Indeed, as Karl Popper argued in his classic work distinguishing science from pseudoscience: if we cannot describe what evidence could count against a theory we are considering, it is not a scientific theory at all, but only a set of beliefs unsupported by evidence.

After showing, in detail, why mathematical models for Earth surface change are irreparably misleading, the Pilkeys conclude:

> . . . not recognizing complexity is what has allowed us to escape from reality through quantitative mathematical modeling . . . It is a world where mathematical equations characterize events and processes, equations that can describe only a small part of the picture in very simple fashion. The intuition of an experienced scientist is gone. At best, only a small fraction of the processes that lead to the desired endpoint prediction can be considered . . . if we wish to stay within the bounds of reality we must look to a more qualitative future, a future where there will be no certain answers to many of the important questions we have . . .

These authors address the challenges of predicting changes in the Earth's surface and illuminate the general difficulties of seeking more precision than current understanding allows. They also recognize the dangers of acting as if we had that precision—or any right to expect it. The complex vagaries of dealing with judicial and medical subjects are no less challenging.

Were I to propose a toast to what the Pilkeys have said, and to their lucidity in saying it, it would be with good wine. There's no reason ever to drink bad wine. It wouldn't have to be great wine, but something that would at least prompt the oenophiles to nod with approval. And we wouldn't want it to be hugely expensive. If price were no object, it would be easy to make a good choice—perhaps the 2004 Charmes-Chambertain at about $400 a bottle. But nearly all of us must keep an eye on the budget. So maybe we would seek the advice of experts, looking to their carefully developed ratings to guide us. Many of us are familiar with the increasingly prominent 100-point rating scales used by leading wine critics, the publications where their work appears, and the merchants and marketers who rely on those ratings. If we see an 82-point wine for $25, we know enough to keep looking. If we see a 94-point wine for $60, most of us still keep looking. And when we see that 91-point wine for $15, we brighten—knowing that we stand before a great opportunity. But it's nonsense. It's a silly dance, and even the choreographers acknowledge that. As the *New York Times* reported, Joshua Greene, editor of *Wine & Spirits*, said, "On many levels it's nonsensical . . . I don't think it's a very valuable piece of information." William Tisherman, former editor of *Wine Enthusiast*, said, "The deeper you get into this, the more you realize how misleading and misguided this all is." And Michael De Loach, of the admirable Hook and Ladder winery—which makes a splendid and reasonable Chardonnay, for example—says, "If Parker or *Spectator* don't give you a high enough score, you can make up your own . . . applying a 100 point scale to wine is dishonest. It makes the consumer think it is scientific." It's the wine world's analogue to Bruun's Rule.

The great English philosopher G. E. Moore, discussing the grounding of moral judgment, gave the name "The Naturalistic

Fallacy" to any attempt to infer what ought to be done from propositions about the natural world, no matter how well substantiated those were. This point of view is often summarized by the aphorism, "You can't derive an '*ought*' from an '*is*.'" There's a long lineage to this perspective, from pre-Socratics such as Protagoras, through the Scottish empiricist David Hume—and they all understood that human values require human judgment to be applied even after all the relevant facts are assembled. Indeed, even the determination of which facts are relevant requires judgment about values.

Such judgments about values are inherently reflected in the framing of the regulations we adopt and in the algorithms that determine what computers do. That is widely understood. The need for evaluative judgment in the implementation and enforcement of regulations is comparably inherent, but far less visible, and we overlook or override that need at our peril. We have an affinity for what can be counted, measured, checked against lists, verified, recorded, reduced to PowerPoint slides, and then defended in a way that protects us from substantive responsibility for our judgments. PowerPoint can work beautifully for visual imagery, such as showing the difference between two kinds of lesions that can easily be mistaken for one another, or for presenting important images in art history, architecture, or costume design, or for dramatically showing how terrifyingly fast the irreversible and deadly retreat of glaciers is, worldwide. Sometimes it is even effective for presenting graphic data, although it is misused far more often than it is useful. (If that seems harsh, see Edward Tufte's persuasive twenty-eight-page monograph called *The Cognitive Style of PowerPoint*. Among the most compelling demonstrations of the distorting limitations of PowerPoint is one reprinted there: Peter Norvig's account of Lincoln's Gettysburg Address, as it would have been had

Lincoln been doing it as a PowerPoint presentation.) It fails at facilitating conceptual clarification, stimulating critical inquiry, and prompting important questions—that is, it fails at contributing to actual, serious thought.

It may be intriguing to discover that there are substantive connections among such ostensibly diverse subjects as cheese shops, baseball umpires, sonnet writers, and all the rest, but that's not enough. What is intriguing is not always important—except perhaps to whomever it intrigues. We must ask finally whether there is any persuasive operational message here. Unsurprisingly, I think so.

We need a Campaign for Responsible Judgment. Bad judgment exists, of course. But the remedy is not to try to exclude judgment. Nor should flawed judgment necessarily be a hanging offense, if it does not flow from venality or from culpable negligence or ineptitude. Here's what I want my readers to do:

1. Sharpen your detectors and ask always whether the matter before you rests on prior judgments that might not bear close scrutiny—or requires new judgments that will.

2. Be on the lookout for the judgment-averse: the ubiquitous, tedious, algorithmic automata who have no sense of the larger purpose that is undermined by their parochial procedural perfectionism. They can do great damage. Remember Wiener's Warning.

3. Determine for yourself what the scope of your role is to be. If you are asked to address a specific question, pause and ask what purpose the question is meant to serve. If you applaud that purpose, ask whether addressing the question in the form in which it was presented to you does serve that purpose.

4. To the extent that you can, view pending decisions through the lens of a Responsible Judgment Advocate. That should be a prelude to an enduring habit of mind. Thus, and finally,

5. In all your roles and dealings, be an active advocate for informed, empirically grounded, responsible, *qualitative* judgment, whenever algorithmic and purely quantitative analyses are inadequate—which is most of the time.

I was asked by a federal agency to join a site-visit team. Three of us, including a program officer from the agency, were lodged at a lovely hotel. Instead of having dinner in the hotel's expensive dining room—which the program officer assured us would be appropriate—we went to a terrific casual ethnic restaurant a few miles away. That cost about one third of what the hotel dinner would have cost. I paid our $4 taxi fare back to the hotel. Later, my request for expense reimbursement was rejected. I had not, in the words of the rejection letter, "documented the unavailability of dinner at the hotel." I replied that the problem was the lack of lodging at the restaurant. Eventually, I got my expenses reimbursed—minus that $4.

I rest my case.

21

A TROLLEY, A CANE, AND GREEN TEA ICE CREAM

Ideas do not exist in a vacuum and thinkers should not be defined merely through their works.

— David Edmonds and John Eidinow,
Rousseau's Dog (2007)

At first glance, Philippa Foot and Marjorie Grene would seem to have little in common. The tall, stately Foot exuded an aura of English aristocracy: calm, elegant, and unflappable. Grene, of Eastern European Jewish heritage, was short, earthy, volcanic, unpredictable. Neither followed a traditional path; each achieved greatness as legendary philosophers—on both sides of the Atlantic—with immense and lasting influence within philosophy and beyond it. I met Philippa in Oxford, where she was a Fellow of Somerville College— Oxford's oldest college for women, named for the inspiring Scottish feminist and brilliant mathematician and scientist

Mary Somerville (1780–1872). We became friends and stayed in touch. In 1976, she began a professorship at UCLA. When I was planning to be in Los Angeles we arranged to have dinner together, and Philippa proposed to pick me up at my hotel. At the appointed hour, a pastel convertible suddenly appeared, top down, the smiling driver looking like something from a "visit Hollywood" advertisement with her stylish hat and large sunglasses. Philippa explained that she'd decided to go all in and be a California Girl while she was there. Off we went to the Hana Sushi restaurant, a favorite of hers near the campus. After some spectacular sushi, Philippa recommended the green tea ice cream. I had never had or even heard of green tea ice cream and timidly declined. She leaned forward and calmly said, "That would be a poor decision. You really should try it." I replied that I would be willing to do so, but at another time. She looked at me intensely for a moment, turned to the server, and said, "We shall have two orders of green tea ice cream." It was marvelous, and I have had it often ever since.

Philippa mentioned an upcoming visit to Washington, D.C., and I asked whether I could assist since I was then at Maryland, in the D.C. area. She said there was one site she would especially like to see: the home where her mother was born. I hadn't known her mother was American. The conversation follows:

> SG: Of course, gladly, if you have the address and if the house is still there. There's been so much redevelopment over the years one can't be certain.

> PF: I'm quite sure it's still there, and I do know the address. It's 1600 Pennsylvania Avenue.

SG: 1600? On Pennsylvania? But I think that's the White House address.

PF: Yes, I understand that's what you call it.

Thus I learned that Philippa's mother was Esther Cleveland, daughter of U.S. president Grover Cleveland, and the only presidential child born in the White House. Esther married Captain William Sidney Bence Bosanquet of the Coldstream Guards, joining the English aristocracy. Esther's sister Ruth (not born in the White House) became known as Baby Ruth, the namesake of a popular candy bar.

One call to the White House sufficed to arrange for Philippa's visit. We even had a parking space awaiting inside the gates, near the front door. As a guide took our small group along a hallway and around a corner, Philippa abruptly pointed to a portrait on the wall, excitedly exclaiming, "Oh, there's grandfather!" It was—the grandfather she never knew, who had died a dozen years before she was born. It seemed to me that she was then a bit embarrassed by suddenly becoming a center of attention herself! Because President Carter was elsewhere, we were taken into the Oval Office. That office appears often in news reports; seeing it always reinforces my gratitude for having been there with Philippa. The heightened security necessitated by the lethal January 6 insurrection, however, makes me wonder what it would take now to arrange such a visit, even with the indomitable Philippa Foot along.

Philippa's childhood was one of wealth, but not privilege. She was raised at Kirkleatham Old Hall, a sixteen-room mansion on fifteen acres in Yorkshire, infused with the mores and practices of the upper crust. Philippa mostly did not go to school, but was tutored by governesses who, on her later account, left her completely uneducated. She was typically presented to her parents at teatime for an hour, but other-wise had scant interaction with them. A bout of abdominal tuberculosis when she was around eight kept her an invalid for the better part of a year. She was isolated and lonely, and before she was twenty she had resolved to escape and find her own way through further education—despite strong opposition from her parents. They thought such ambitions were inappropriate for a girl of her breeding and station. And yet she became one of the giants of philosophy—with on-going positions at Oxford and UCLA, in countless appear-ances elsewhere, and through the influence of her work on philosophy, economics, law, political science, religion, and more. Philippa kept that position at UCLA for fifteen years, dividing her time between Los Angles and Britain.

I met Marjorie Grene through the Council for Philo-sophical Studies (whose programs I administered for several years). She was born in 1910 in Milwaukee, where her father, Harry Glicksman, was a professor of English at the University of Wisconsin-Milwaukee. Marjorie was therefore just approach-ing her teenage years when the 19th Amendment was ratified on August 18, 1920. Her mother, Edna Kerngood Glicksman, became a leader in the Wisconsin League of Women Voters, so feminist values were part of Marjorie's lineage. She had a promising academic start, with an undergraduate degree in zoology from Wellesley and a doctorate in philosophy from Radcliffe. But positions in philosophy were rare, and rarer still for women, so she had to take what she could find. She spent several years at the University of Chicago, where her schol-ar-farmer husband, the classicist David Grene, was co-founder of the Committee on Social Thought. But her untenured posi-tion ended in 1944, and she interrupted her formal academic life for fifteen years. She was then a farmer and mother, also on both sides of the Atlantic, but despite those demands kept writing important philosophical works all the while. By the time I met her, she, like Philippa, was acclaimed as a pioneering philosopher of immense distinction and influence within and beyond the field. On the occasion of her receiving an award from the American Philosophical Association, Alasdair MacIntyre (author of *After Virtue*, mentioned earlier, and my co-author on an article about medical fallibility) said, approximately, "The traditional philosopher is expected to follow an argument wherever it leads. Marjorie tells it where it damn well had better go!"

Marjorie, too, had a faculty appointment at the University of California, hers at the Davis campus. When she was sixty-three, severe trouble with a knee limited her mobility, so she went to an orthopedic specialist in San Francisco. She recounted the conversation to me:

> Dr: Well, you *are* sixty-three, and knees deteriorate with age.
>
> MG: Young Man, I know perfectly well what my age is. Need I point out to you that my *right* knee, which does *not* trouble me, like my left knee is also sixty-three years old, and it is the difference between them, and not their age, that I am paying you these *exorbitant* fees to discover.

That sounded just like Marjorie, and I had a twinge of sympathy for the doc, whose training probably did not equip him adequately to go toe to toe with Professor Grene! Somehow, she told me later, the knee problem diminished, and I was pleased that her mobility increased. So I was surprised when, on meeting her at the Washington airport, I saw her using a cane. I asked about the knee.

MG: Oh, the knee is better. But I learned that
people are ever so much kinder to old ladies
using a cane, so I always use it going through
any airport.

When Marjorie died at ninety-eight in 2009, she had
essentially created the field of philosophy of biology, changed
how evolutionary theory is understood, and redirected
much philosophical and scientific thinking through her
thirteen books and a practice, in the words of her colleague
Richard Burian, of "bucking the mainstream of philosophical thought for her entire career." She didn't, as MacIntyre
quipped, merely tell specific arguments where to go. She told
the whole field of philosophy of science—and it went.

Philippa was born on October 3, 1920, twelve years to
the day after my mother Della's birth. And Philippa died on
October 3, 2010, her own ninetieth birthday. As scholars, the
long-lived Foot and Grene transformed their fields. Della
wrote nothing, but as a teacher she changed lives. She retired
as a beloved and acclaimed sixth-grade teacher in Brookline,
Massachusetts, at seventy. As a widow in her eighties, she
moved to an apartment in a continuing care community near
Boston. No longer constrained by my father's extremely narrow culinary preferences, she became an octogenarian gastronomic adventurer. I delighted in taking her, at her request,
for her first sushi, Indian, and Thai meals. Philippa would not
have had to ask her twice to try the green tea ice cream.

In that living environment, Della plunged into their cultural, intellectual, and governance activities, with special
interest in helping staff improve their education. A bonus
for me was having many opportunities to give guest lectures
there to an enthusiastic, well-prepared, and energetic audience. But time took its toll; she eventually lost the ability to

live in that apartment and moved into assisted living at age ninety-eight. Many staff there were immigrants; she helped them with vocabulary and pronunciation, making flash cards to aid the tutoring. A few others were part-time students, and they brought her drafts of their papers, which she helped edit. She was still an eager learner and dedicated teacher.

Two years later, in October 2008, I took what are among my most treasured pictures of her, microphone in hand, addressing a large gathering of admirers and expressing her surprise at being able to welcome them to her one-hundredth birthday party. Shortly after that, her health declined. The election of 2008 was imminent. She asked me to get an absentee ballot for her, as she was not able to vote at the polls. In my naivete, I said "Mom, you don't have to be concerned about that. Obama has a sixty-point lead in Massachusetts." A superb teacher to the very end, she swiftly set me straight, saying this had nothing to do with the outcome. She said, "This is an important moment in American history and I want to know I have been part of it." I did as she asked, and she voted for Obama. Six months later, she was gone. As we think about the very elderly, we should always be mindful of what they can teach us and of how easily we can overlook what matters to them in ways we can and must support. There's a saying perhaps of African origin and endorsed within our Native American communities that I wish were embraced by our entire culture: "When we lose an elder, it is as if a library has burned down."

How to think about the frail and declining elderly is a frequent topic in bioethics. Discussions about it are pervasively influenced by Philippa's classic work on "the trolley problem." In its simplest version, the trolley problem posits the following situation: you are at the switch of a trolley line that has left and right branches. Stuck on the left branch are five immobilized people (never mind why) and on the right branch is one stuck person. The switch is set for the trolley to keep left, surely killing five. You could flip the switch to the right, killing one person to save five. Or, unwilling to cause the death of an innocent person, you could do nothing. What should you do?

Students typically try to skirt the problem by seeking a technical fix. Isn't there a way to stop the trolley? Maybe some of the people could be unbound? What if you could warn them? Once that avoidance behavior is set aside, the tough moral challenge remains. Would it matter if the one on the right had saved your life, was your mother, or was a famous young scientist at the start of a brilliant career? Would it matter if the five were a student basketball team, a gang escaped from prison, or five first responders who had been rushing to the scene of a trolley accident? As soon as we ask what the morally relevant factors are, we face fundamental issues in ethics, including the question of whether there is a legitimate distinction between actively killing someone and letting someone die by not taking an action we could have taken. It's a short step to a medical analogue: One healthy young person recovering well from elective surgery and five nearby patients facing death due to the failure of a (different) vital organ. Why not sacrifice the one in order to save five by gently easing the healthy patient into a painless coma and harvesting the five organs for transplant? Would it matter if the healthy patient, as a committed utilitarian, agreed to that sacrifice? Or even had proposed it? Philippa's trolley has arrived in the hospital, delivering the challenge to confront our assumptions and convictions about utilitarian choices versus other kinds of moral values. We are soon probing matters of precedent, trust, role responsibility, consent, and more. This was at issue in my conversations with the reporter, recounted in Chapter 8, about the allocation of ventilators during the early days of the Covid pandemic. He thought it obvious that utilitarian values should dominate but had no awareness of how difficult it is to understand what outcomes are most likely, even apart from the significance of non-utilitarian values.

The Syracuse Philosophy Department has a small seminar and library room, with a fine view to the north, shelves containing several hundred philosophy books, and pictures of thirteen famous philosophers. One is of Philippa Foot. I've no idea how many of the hundreds of students who have been in that room ever noticed the pictures or recognized their subjects if they have. But nearly all of them would know of Philippa's intellectual importance—unaware that her grandfather, an American president, had lived just twenty minutes away at 109 Academy Street in Fayetteville.

Philippa was not a mother; the childhood tuberculosis left her unable to bear children, as she learned only several years after her marriage. (She and Michael Foot divorced shortly after that sad discovery.) Marjorie's two children each achieved great academic distinction. Nicholas Grene, a renowned scholar of English literature, was head of the English Department at Trinity College, Dublin, and is now emeritus. Ruth Grene, a pre-eminent scholar in plant biology and bioinformatics, is professor emerita at Virginia Tech. Both Ruth and Nicholas have children so two generations now trace their lineage back to Marjorie.

Ruth is an active force for reducing the continuing manifestations of racial injustice that remain powerful throughout our culture. (By odd coincidence, I write these words on June 19th, 2002, the Juneteenth national holiday celebrating the resilience and durability of America's African Americans, their essential and undervalued contributions to the building of the nation, and the immense agenda of unfinished business on the path to a just society.)

An interest in philosophy draws us to the philosophers whose work connects most strongly with that initial interest. As we study their work and follow it where it takes us, we sometimes become interested in the lives of those philosophers and what led and enabled them to do that work. We want to know about the struggles they faced, the barriers they overcame, the help they received, the compromises they made. These three women—Marjorie, Philippa, and Della—two philosophers and a teacher of children, each became a strong, admired, influential and independent-minded professional despite the constraining and distressing circumstances of their era.

My father finished law school in 1929, just in time for the Great Depression. In my parents' early years, frugality was imprinted on them. For my mother, it was so ingrained that, although always generous to others, it would never have occurred to her to spend money self-indulgently, for example, on fancy clothes or jewelry. In her most advanced years, we typically left restaurants with small containers of leftovers; she thought it unacceptable to waste food by leaving it behind. Those containers remained in her freezer until I tossed them to make room for later ones.

Marjorie became unsympathetic to the logical positivist perspective that was made widely visible by AJ Ayer in his *Language, Truth, and Logic* (1936), in which he advocated modeling philosophy after what he saw as the objective, empirically rigorous sciences. She had already studied that perspective at Radcliffe with C. I. Lewis. Whereas Philippa's concern was focused sharply on moral philosophy, Marjorie roamed around the philosophical landscape, historical and

European as well as British, before ultimately focusing on the philosophy of biology with an emphasis on evolution and Darwinism.

Philippa struggled with the prevailing Oxford view that unlike facts, supportable or refutable by evidence, values were just expressions of preference or exhortations to act in one way or another, and thus could never justifiably be called erroneous. She could not accept such perspectives but didn't see how to defeat them. Learning of the Holocaust was transformative for her: it was unthinkable that one could not condemn the Nazis as objectively evil, "absolutely wicked," as she told Jonathan Ree in a BBC interview. Figuring out how to defend that condemnation became the focus of her work, which redirected moral philosophy.

Shortly after the end of the war in 1945, J. L. Austin, the pillar of "ordinary language" analysis and another opponent of logical positivism, began to host regular Saturday morning meetings of the brightest philosophical minds in his orbit. As he was the oldest of the group, it became known as Austin's Kindergarten. As Philippa explained to Ree: "Everyone was asked who had any teaching post in Oxford but the women were not asked. That was a place where work was being done."

These women are part of a lineage with a richly complex past and a future they could not likely have imagined. Thus it is for us all. As we learn about their lives, as well as their work, we learn about ourselves and can think more deeply about the past we carry with us and the future we hope will follow.

22

PERFECTION, REJECTION, AND EXPECTATION

Even if you're a .300 hitter, you're going to fail at your job seven out of ten times.

—Ted Williams *The Science of Hitting* (1970)

A midterm progress report is purely diagnostic, to support student progress. It has no bearing on grades, but merely informs both student and professor about how well prepared the student is at that point in the term. It can indicate strengths and correctable weaknesses in the student's understanding. Before that midterm report was due, I gave my class a practice examination—one that showed what the questions would be like on a real exam. Then I let them see the best answers to each question as written by their classmates. That practice exam also guided what I should indicate in the midterm progress report. Directly after those reports were released, a trembling, tearful student astonished me by claiming that she had been harmed by the midterm report, thought it unfair, and asked how it could be appealed.

> SG: But your practice exam was one of the best in the class, and your midterm report said you were doing "A" quality work. Why are you upset?
>
> Student: My parents reward me when a final grade shows improvement over the midterm report. You made that impossible. I can't improve over an "A."
>
> SG: So you want a *lower* grade on your midterm report?
>
> Student: Yes, please.

I don't recall how I handled this challenge, but I wouldn't have revised an accurate report already sent. I hope I found ways to help the student gain more independence, a healthier understanding of expectations, and a less destructive relationship with her parents.

In our interactions with students there are always voices and experiences in the background that influence how we feel, what we hear, and how we decide. That applies also between physicians and patients; thus the classic medical aphorism, "Who the patient is, is as important as what the patient has." Part of who a patient, student, or faculty member *is* can include parents, influential peers, mentors, past traumatic experiences, economic stressors such as food insecurity, confusion about performance evaluation, and many other factors. My conversation with the student who protested her midterm report called to mind a prior conversation in Palo Alto.

Bob Scott had been an accomplished sociologist at Princeton before becoming associate director of the Center for Advanced Studies in Behavioral Sciences at Stanford. Visiting him there, I learned of his distress about a student who was, he said, among the few best sociology students he had ever had. Her parents were resolved that she would become a physician or lawyer, never praised her accomplishments, but reacted severely to any deviation from perfection. Her becoming a lawyer or physician would be acceptable to them; pursuing her love of sociology would not. Bob had asked her, "If those careers would be just 'acceptable' for you, what do you think it would take for them to praise what you've done?" She paused, shrugged her shoulders, and replied sadly, "Having my own country." This same theme is explored effectively in Pixar's gorgeous animated film *Turning Red* (2022), in which the protagonist, Meilin Lee, is a teen-aged girl struggling to overcome the internalized expectations of an overbearing perfectionist mother.

Sometimes our role as educators requires helping students recalibrate their aspirations by expanding their awareness of the possible. For Scott's student, it was essential that she become able to use her considerable talents in gratifying ways without feelings of guilt or inadequacy based on disapproval by others. Helping her redirect her aspirations was required. Sometimes, the recalibration takes a different form. In our Linked Lenses class, my co-teacher Cathryn Newton and I had a student (AK) whose explicit aspiration was to do well enough to get into a medical school. Early in the term Newton asked to discuss what to do about AK. I had not seen any problem, but Newton explained that AK's aspirations were far too limited and we had to help her understand that. So we worked with her that term and throughout her undergraduate years, emphasizing that we were reliable at spotting future stars who were not aiming high enough. In her senior year she was offered many fully funded spots in M.D.-Ph.D. programs, including top tier schools. She now has both degrees, an impressive funding and publication record, and—still young—is a nationally recognized force in her field. We've recently reminded her that we were right to insist that she'd do well enough to get into medical school!

Spotting talent like that is a judgmental art; there's no systematic way of doing it, whether you're nurturing students, baseball players, or animated filmmakers. MIT became a focus of national debate because of its reintroduction of SAT-ACT test requirements as one among many application factors. The university defended its position on the grounds that "There is no path through MIT that does not rest on a rigorous foundation in mathematics, and we need to be sure our students are ready for that as soon as they arrive." In the same week that MIT announced that decision, *Breaking Ranks* (2022), by Colin Divers—former president of Reed College—provided a scathing critique of college, university, and law school rankings, arguing that standardized tests obscure rather than illuminate the potential for success of individual students.

Just as spotting talent is a judgmental art, so is helping students gain better insight into what their talents are. I'm thrilled by Ketanji Brown Jackson's confirmation as a Supreme Court Justice. But some well-intended reactions are distressing. U.S. District Court Judge Charles Fleming, in Cleveland, praising the inspirational power of her confirmation, said:

> Children of all backgrounds can see that whatever it is that you want to do, if you work hard, if you study, if you put in the time, you can do and you can be anything you want to do or be.

It's not true. We all have limitations that no amount of work, study, and time can overcome. We don't want students to undervalue their capacities, but neither should we want them to embrace grandiose expectations that foretell failure. By Fleming's account, one who fails to achieve a desired goal is responsible for that failure—due to insufficient work, study, or time. That's a prescription for unwarranted feelings of guilt, when so many failures are due to none of the above. Fleming's failure to meet my expectations for rigor and clarity in Federal judges is likely due to an excess of exuberance and an insufficient suspicion of pernicious platitudes. I'm sure he works and studies hard for prodigious amounts of time.

The quest for perfection has a further danger. Achieving a long-sought goal flawlessly can be devastating. This is elegantly described in Jazmina Barrera's *On Lighthouses* (2020); she recounts the fatal desperation of David Foster Wallace following his majestic 1079-page masterpiece, *Infinite Jest* (1996):

> It should be no surprise that once Foster Wallace had handed in the manuscript, he lost his sense of purpose. What would be his last novel, *The Pale King*, wasn't meeting his expectations. He was afraid that perfection had been granted him once and only once . . . . The ultimate attainment of the desired object is unbearable: it annuls motivation, annihilates meaning.

A high school friend's father was a prosperous MIT alumnus, determined that his son also go to MIT. He reluctantly applied, but, with inadequate credentials, was rejected. The insistent father then enrolled him elsewhere for a year of remediation, made donations to MIT, and saw his tenacious insistence pay off when a new application was successful. The son enrolled at MIT, but as a result of such a clear mismatch he was gone after one painful term. It's not that he "wasn't smart." He was very smart and has achieved great success in business and significant philanthropy. He just wasn't smart in the specific ways that MIT required, such as possessing a ready command of basic tools of mathematical analysis. Pressuring him to meet someone else's expectations obscured and suppressed the flourishing of his talents, such as the ability to connect respectfully with people in all walks of life, to think creatively about business opportunities, to muster the resources and people to turn ideas into products—and to be willing to take risks and acknowledge failures without distress.

Students who have not dealt with rejection are ill-prepared for what lies ahead. The quest for perfection can be acceptable with the understanding that there will be instructive failures along the way, including perhaps painful rejections. Without that understanding, the quest is limiting and destructive. I've had one marvelous job after another; I don't know of anyone luckier. But I was rejected by most of the jobs I applied for, sometimes in appallingly insensitive ways. I was even rejected by one for which I had not applied! (Among my treasures is a letter from the head of the search committee for the chancellorship of the University of Illinois at Urbana-Champaign, regretting to inform me that a few final candidates were advanced for interviews, but I was not among them. I had never been a candidate; that letter was the only communication I ever had about that search. I drafted a reply that, as Scribe for the Bethesda-Chevy Chase Dining and Debate Society, it was my duty to inform him that after a thorough consideration of his attributes, we voted without dissent that he was unfit to be invited to join. I enjoy writing such letters; I don't send them.)

Our choices are pervaded by expectations—those we have of ourselves, those we have of others, those we believe others have of us—and by how we respond to those expectations. It's easy to be misled, confused, or discouraged amidst this swirl of perceptions. Avoiding the pitfalls by making good judgments about expectations is a sophisticated art, well worth cultivating with all the intellectual and emotional honesty we have. Long ago, Paul Goodman wrote *Growing Up Absurd* (1960). It was rejected by nineteen publishers, who saw no market for such a radical contrarian screed. I had the opportunity to ask him how he persisted after so many rejections. He replied that he had unwavering confidence in the work and a belief that eventually someone would see its merits. Random House eventually did; at the time of our conversation the paperback edition had sold about 100,000 copies, on its way to half a million. That story sustained me years later when I struggled past many rejections to find a publisher for *Moral Problems in Medicine* (see Chapter 9).

When Matt Diffee, mentioned earlier, spoke with our *Linked Lenses* students, he emphasized that 90 percent of his cartoon submissions to the *New Yorker* were rejected. Professor Newton noted that this is an excellent metaphor for working in science. With many students conditioned to expect to "get the answer right," it takes repeated efforts to open their minds to the idea that the pursuit of knowledge is inherently flawed, requiring tenacious commitment to recurrent corrections, reconsiderations, and renewed efforts, and that their expectations should be commensurate with that reality.

Creative accomplishments are typically like that in all fields. We ought to reject the expectation of perfection on the part of others—and of ourselves.

CHANGING OUR MINDS

There was never a night or a problem that could defeat sunrise or hope.

—Bernard Williams

Bernard Arthur Owens Williams was, by all accounts, among the few most influential philosophers of his time. In his obituary in *The Guardian* (June 13, 2003), Jane O'Grady wrote: "Arguably the greatest British philosopher of his era, he brought wit and compassion to the moral questions of society." Being in his presence was like experiencing an intellectual fireworks display. His mentor, Gilbert Ryle—among the most influential Oxford philosophers—said of Williams, "He understands what you're going to say better than you understand it yourself, and sees all the possible objections to it, and all the possible answers to all the possible objections, before you've got to the end of your own sentence."

Once Bernard and I drove from Haverford, Pennsylvania, to Maryland, and he delighted in reading aloud the roadside signs naming each municipality we passed through, large or small, along that 135-mile journey. When we arrived, he said he had enjoyed seeing them, and recited most of their names in the order of our route. When I gave a lecture at King's College in Cambridge at his invitation, he was provost and lived in the Provost's Lodge adjacent to King's College Chapel. At times, he did ceremonial readings there—his deep, resonant voice a perfect match for the glorious gothic surroundings. At times his young sons played in that chapel, which they considered a perquisite of living next door.

Bernard agreed to speak at the University of Maryland. I asked for a copy of his CV so I could prepare to introduce him properly. He did not have it readily available, but said he'd have his assistant send it. I reminded him before I left; he promised to do it. He didn't. I called from Maryland, emphasizing that time was running out. Finally, I called one last time and said that if I did not receive his CV, I would make one up as I saw fit and introduce him based on that. And I did. With Bernard in the front row, I called the session to order and said:

> Bernard Williams first came to the attention of the British public when he was abandoned as an infant in the Underground station at Tooting Bec, where his plaintive wails echoed resoundingly from the station's tile walls, thus inducing his well-known, life-long love of opera.

I continued in that vein for a few moments, then called him to the podium. Completely unfazed, he thanked me for my generous introduction and began his lecture. That earned him an honorarium, for which I had to complete forms affirming that he had done what he was engaged to do, after which the request would be processed and I would eventually receive a check to mail to him. I regretted that slow bureaucratic procedure; the gracious way to treat a guest speaker is to present the honorarium during the visit. I had often appreciated such graciousness, had also experienced long delays, and once even had an honorarium rescinded because the sponsors took exception to part of my presentation. I resolved to treat my future guests properly.

When Charles Fried, solicitor general of the United States, came to Syracuse University, I had his honorarium check ready in advance. Before introducing him to the audience, I told him the following:

> Charles, I've known you long enough and well enough to be confident that you're not the kind of guy who will leave as soon as you have your honorarium, whether you've spoken or not. So here it is, and I really look forward to hearing what you have to say.

He thanked me and slipped the envelope into his jacket pocket. He then presented his talk, "The Courts and the Constitution: Federalism, Separation of Powers, and Constitutionalism." After much lively conversation with the audience, as I was thanking him for the session, he reclaimed the microphone and added one last comment: "As solicitor general, I am barred by law from accepting payment for any speeches I give. So, with my thanks, I return this to you." And with a grand, courtly flourish, he handed the envelope back to me.

In those days, Charles was a staunch Republican, conservative across a broad range of issues. In the Trump era, his views evolved to the point that he actively supported Biden for president. He told me recently that he is close to completing

a new book on metanoia (a transformative change of heart).
I replied:

> I'll be fascinated to hear about this. A classic
> example I suppose is Ashoka [268—232 BCE],
> whose bloody rule of India gave way to a com-
> mitment to nonviolence. Would a more recent
> example be Fried, now cheering for that newer
> Indian, Katyal, and supporting Biden despite
> being historically a Republican?

Neal Katyal had been acting solicitor general in the Obama
administration and is well known for progressive, liberal
Democratic views. Charles pointed out that he now agrees
with Neal's positions on Constitutional matters and has even
filed amicus briefs in support of Neal's efforts. Katharine
Whitehorn had said, "The wind of change, whatever it is, blows
most freely through an open mind." I applauded Charles's
open mind and his own metanoia, adding that I'd been at
both of Neal's weddings. This startled Charles, who thought
Neal had been married only once. I explained that Neal's
bride Joanna Rosen was Jewish. At Joanna's parents' bucolic
property in Saugerties, NY, on a blazing hot summer morning,
there was a typical Jewish wedding. Then, following a lavish
lunch interval that included the complete restructuring of the
setting, there was a second wedding. Neal—as a traditional
Indian groom, veiled and arriving on a white horse—was
married to Joanna again. Two weddings, despite that first
assumption, did not mean two wives. Charles was gleeful at
this revelation of a difference between appearance and reality,
and he readily changed his mind about Neal's marital history.

"What would it take to get you to change your mind?" I put this
question to students in every course, often drawing on Charles

Sanders Peirce's classic article "The Fixation of Belief"(1877), in which he considers the various ways people come to have the beliefs they have, reviews the advantages of each, and endorses the scientific method as most favorable because it alone invites revision—changing one's mind—in light of new evidence. He knew the wind of change blows most easily through an open mind. Most of the students, when pressed, acknowledge formerly believing in the existence of Santa Claus, but they no longer do so. We then explore the origins of that belief and the processes by which it was shed. This leads to distinguishing between a belief like that—not essential to their sense of who and what they are—and their core beliefs, ones far harder to relinquish without disrupting their world view. To cease believing in Santa Claus is part of growing up. To disavow white supremacy and become an active advocate of anti-racism, as people like Chris Buckley and Arno Michaelis have done, is metanoia.

I want the students to adopt the practice of asking, for any belief under consideration, where on that spectrum it belongs, and why—and of reassessing the belief in light of that reflection. That's not an easy practice to apply and overdoing it can be immobilizing. Everything we do, all day long, springs from some combination of our beliefs and our motivations; we can't scrutinize our beliefs all along the way and get anything done. But when a belief is challenged or is foundational to some position we take on an important and controversial matter, an honest inquiry into the basis for that belief can be affirming or transforming. That's hard work. I want the students to practice doing it, because the need for it can arise unexpectedly at any time. It's the sort of skill that grows with practice, as does an awareness that such inquiries help us understand our own values more deeply. I want the students to sharpen their ability to detect those times when probing their own values is appropriate, and to increase their confidence that they know how to do it. I'd like you to do that, too.

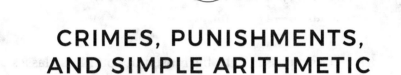

24

CRIMES, PUNISHMENTS, AND SIMPLE ARITHMETIC

My object all sublime, I shall achieve in time, To let the punishment fit the crime, The punishment fit the crime; And make each prisoner pent, Unwillingly represent, A source of innocent merriment. Of innocent merriment!

—W. S. Gilbert and A. Sullivan, *The Mikado* (1885)

In Dostoevsky's *Crime and Punishment* (1866), Raskolnikov—an impoverished student brooding over his plight and that of other destitute people—contemplates the wealth of an elderly, corrupt, distasteful woman to whom he is financially beholden. In a tavern, he overhears another student expressing similar concerns about that same woman:

> Look here; on one side we have a stupid, sense-
> less, worthless, spiteful, ailing, horrid old

woman, not simply useless but doing actual mischief, who has no idea what she is living for herself . . . On the other side, fresh young lives thrown away for want of help and by thousands, on every side! A hundred thousand good deeds could be done and helped, on that old woman's money which will be buried in a monastery! One death, and a hundred lives in exchange—it's simple arithmetic!

This classic passage has been used in countless classes to raise questions of ethics, law, religion, social justice, and more. It was used in an *Introduction to Ethics* course taught by Donald Davidson (you met him in Chapter 9), for whom I was one of two teaching assistants. Each student submitted a short essay about that passage. As I sat in my office grading their papers, I was interrupted by the other TA who burst in saying "Listen to this one!" And he read "No amount of good can outweigh the nearly infinite value of a human life." We laughed heartily at the absurdity of the phrase "nearly infinite" and agreed that some linguistic therapy about numbers and counting was urgently needed by that student. I graded several more papers, and then read "No amount of good can outweigh the nearly infinite value of a human life." I raced to the other TA's office with that paper in hand. We compared the two essays; they were identical.

The students assumed that because their papers would be seen by different TAs, the dishonesty would be unde-tectable. They had not foreseen the forensic fortuity of their linguistic lapse. We informed Davidson right away; he told us to say nothing about it to the students, to retain their papers, and to leave the matter to him. In the next meeting of the class, as he discussed moral choice and the difficulty of anticipating consequences accurately, he gradually worked his way toward the Raskolnikov example, the students' essays, and the unlikely possibility that two students might submit duplicate essays, thinking, perhaps wrongly, that there would be no risk because the papers would be read by different people. But unforeseen consequences are an inherent problem for a Utilitarian approach (acting to produce the best consequences) because, as Hume explained, the future might not conform to the past, and we can never be sure what outcomes our actions will cause. Submitting duplicate papers, Davidson continued, illustrates this general point most usefully. Seated in the back of the room, I could not see the face of my student, nor did I know the other student except by name. But I thought of the well-known (and often misunderstood) boiling frog metaphor, according to which a frog in cold water that is gradually heated a degree at a time will eventually be a boiled frog. I was nearly tempted to feel a tinge of sympathy for these two students. One paper and two TAs is nothing like one bride and two weddings.

This was not the first time I had seen Davidson use his theatrical skills to deal with a student of whom he disapproved. A required course in the first semester for doctoral students was the "Proseminar" in which each new student gave a talk about his or her philosophical interests, followed by a grilling from the faculty. Assessment of the student's prospects was based both on the content of the talk and the student's ability to cope with a rigorous critical onslaught. Davidson's questions were typically the most incisive and challenging. As I've mentioned, of the eighteen new students in that entering class, only five completed the doctorate. But one did not even complete the first term. He gave his Proseminar presentation on the philosophical significance of extra-sensory perception, after which Davidson stood, looked at him intensely, slowly turned away, and silently walked out of the room. That student dropped out promptly thereafter. He got the message that he was not going to survive in the program; the rest of us learned that Davidson was capable of unforgettable cruelty when displeased. We all knew that a private, gentle, and honest advising conversation could have redirected our classmate constructively. We wondered whether the crushing public humiliation was meant somehow to signal something to the rest of us, without regard to its effect on that one student. Seventeen students placed on high alert, one discarded. Simple arithmetic.

Yet arithmetic is often less simple than it seems. Benjamin Oluwakayode Osuntokun was an elegant, patrician Nigerian neurologist whose clinical research on ataxic neuropathy brought international acclaim. At a meeting in Geneva, he told us this: He was treating a patient in Nigeria who had been gravely ill but was recovering well. Ben had to go to London for a week but assured his patient that all would be fine if he complied with medical instructions, taking one dose of medicine with each meal. The patient agreed. Osuntokun returned to find the patient near death. Puzzled, he asked "Have taken all your medicine as instructed?"

Patient: Oh, yes, Doctor, one with each meal.

Doctor: You are sure, three pills every day?

Patient: No, Sir. Just one with each meal. I'm a very poor man, I can only afford to eat once a day.

Ben told us about this to illustrate how easily our familiar assumptions can thwart effective communications. In this case, he assumed three when the reality was one, and that erroneous counting nearly cost a life. The story again under-scores the need to know who the patient is, not just what the patient has.

Ben's story reminded me of a legendary event at Syracuse University that occurred before my arrival. A professor labored mightily to prepare meticulously crafted lectures for his Introduction to Philosophy students. He wrote them in longhand and brought them to class in a binder from which he read each lecture verbatim, rarely looking up from the notes. This was fully in the tradition of the most dreadful Oxford pedagogy. On the day in question, a few minutes into his reading of the lecture, a student interrupted, pointing out that this same lecture had been presented at the previous class. The professor, without the proper notes at hand, simply said "Class dismissed" and left the lecture hall. He had top marks for getting the subject matter precisely right but was a dismal failure at the more important task of getting it across.

Davidson was unsurpassed both at getting the content right and at getting it across. He could also be, as in Gilbert and Sullivan's *Mikado*, a Lord High Executioner. In the case of the two cheating students, the punishment perhaps was appropriate, and I confess to admiring how he boiled those two frogs. But in the Proseminar, the punishment did not fit the crime and there was no merriment. One might even see how the punishment was meted out as something of a crime itself.

Each of these disparate stories is about communicating to one or more audiences. The message as received is not always as intended by the sender, and the audiences are not always what one expects. Whether one is speaking to a class, a patient, an advisee, a companion at a table in a tavern—or submitting an essay—one ought first be clear about what message one wants to convey, and to whom, and then about how that message might be received by intended and unintended receivers, and what all that listening or reading might prompt in consequence of the message. That's a lot to figure out.

Another thread through these stories is the question of what counts when we are counting something. Recall Philippa Foot's field-transforming perception (see Chapter 21) that the holocaust demonstrated the impossibility of basing moral judgment on the time and culture within which events occur. If some events are inherently wrong on qualitative grounds that transcend any calculation of plusses and minuses, we need to probe what grounds do count, and why. Foot pursued that inquiry without recourse to theological assumptions, infusing moral philosophy with new energy and direction. (Recall the related discussions in Chapter 4.)

It may well be that a feminist perspective like hers, focusing qualitatively on the lives of real people rather than on a more sterile attempt to quantify and measure, will lead to deeper understanding of what should count as just, fair, or right. That arithmetic is never simple.

25

TAR PITS, LIME QUARRIES, AND HUMANITY

Only our peaceable instincts make us human. The snarling of hate and the brandishing of weapons is what diminishes us.

—Theodore Bikel, *Theo: An Autobiography* (1994)

When Theodore Bikel died on July 21, 2015, the *New York Times*, in one of its longest obituaries, described him as "a multi-lingual troubadour, character actor, and social activist." Having been in *The African Queen, The Sound of Music,* and *My Fair Lady,* and dominating the stage as Tevya in *Fiddler on the Roof,* he was that, and much more. He was a voracious reader, a serious scholar, an elegant writer, a playwright, a tenacious advocate for his deeply held conviction that every person deserves respect as an equally valuable member of the human community, and a dear friend. The obituary described him as "a bulky bearish man." That he was; he loved good food and tucked into it with great enthusiasm.

I was in Los Angeles to meet with a curator at the Page Museum at the La Brea Tar Pits, as arranged by my colleague Cathryn Newton—an acclaimed paleontologist as well as a renowned oceanographer, and also a close friend of Theo. Not knowing whether he was even in town, given how often he traveled, I thought he might be available for a chat over coffee or some other connection. When I called his cell phone, his wife Aimee answered. That was immediately puzzling. I explained why I was calling, and Aimee said she had answered because they were in the cardiac ICU—to which Theo had been rushed days earlier. He was hooked up to various IV lines and restricted to a liquid diet, which he loathed. As she explained this, I could hear him in the background asking who was on the phone and about what. She told him, they talked briefly, and then she said, "Theo says he knows it's a lot to ask, but if it were possible for you to look in on him here in the hospital, he would welcome that."

"Of course," I said. "I'll be there." The museum wasn't going anywhere; that could be rescheduled. (It was; the image of wooly mammoth tusks on the cover is from the central hall in that museum.) But for all I knew this might be my last chance to visit with Theo, whose condition sounded so fragile. I set out on Highway 10 toward the hospital in Santa Monica, ten terror-filled miles away, as harrowing a road as the wild west offers. It seemed that, should I survive, I would as likely be an admitted patient as a visitor. But despite the clenched teeth, white knuckles, and stress of being surrounded by high-speed careening maniacs, I made it. I entered Theo's room not knowing what to expect.

There he was—bedridden, with IV lines and monitors amidst the trappings of his ICU imprisonment. But far from being dour, he had an indomitable sparkle in his eyes. He said, "Sam, how kind of you to come see me in the hospital! I used to fantasize about starlets. Now I fantasize about applesauce." And there was merriment in the room. I left hoping that he would pull through, but still worried. Two weeks later he was in New York City, performing.

Among Theo's passions was the importance of seeing the commonality in all people, whatever groups they might be in. This requires seeing more deeply than what is apparent on the surface; it's a "sharpening your detectors" point. Reflecting on Theo's life and legacy, I recalled what I had written about Nelson Mandela, published on December 5, 2013—the day of his death:

> The death of Nelson Mandela should prompt us all to reflect on the extraordinary and enduring power of his life.
>
> Years ago I stood in the prison on Robben Island, gripping the bars and looking into the tiny cell where he lived for 18 years—the cell Barack Obama visited recently. The tour guide had explained the humiliations and deprivations of Mandela's long imprisonment, but what seemed beyond explaining is the strength of character that enabled a man to endure such things for so long and then to emerge as a national leader possessed of optimism, generosity of spirit, and a commitment to reconciliation rather than revenge. How is this possible?
>
> When Nazi survivor Elie Wiesel spoke to the first-year students in Syracuse University's College of Arts and Sciences, he emphasized

that hatred is as poisonous when one faces one's tormentors as at any other time. Like Mandela, Wiesel suffered unfathomable personal losses that could easily have crushed his spirit or bred a blazing vindictiveness. Yet each of these men became a force for the power of love, tolerance, respect for difference—for the joy of human potential even in the face of dreadful human realities.

Here is some of what I learned about how Mandela did it: On Robben Island, just outside Table Bay at Cape Town, South Africa, there's a lime quarry. In the brilliant sun, its white walls glare with painful brightness. Mandela, and the other prisoners forced to work long hours there, were not allowed dark glasses. The fine lime dust from their back-breaking work pervaded their clothes, invaded their lungs, irritated their squinting eyes. Some of them, like Mandela, were educated men who knew that even as their bodies labored and suffered, their minds were free and strong. But many other prisoners were uneducated— even illiterate. So the quarry became a place of teaching and learning.

Writing in the dust with sticks, the educated prisoners brought a reverence for the power of knowledge to those who had never had the opportunity to develop their minds. Even prisoners who were criminals, rather than political prisoners, came to understand that grinding poverty, discrimination, ignorance, and lack of opportunity—the wellsprings of crime—were best addressed by empowering their own minds. Some of them became students, too.

This happened before the watchful eyes of prison guards, many of whom were untutored louts. Yet, louts though they were, they saw something valuable that attracted them more than it threatened them. So they also became students, and Mandela and the others taught them out of respect for their humanity and their interest in learning. Those guards experienced affirmations both of mind and of heart—in sharing their knowledge, the educated prisoners displayed a generosity of spirit that prompted both admiration and growing respect from the guards.

For Mandela this was an early stage of the movement toward reconciliation. We marvel at the tenacity and endurance of Ernest Shackleton, whose failed Antarctic exploration in 1914 threatened the lives of his 21 stranded crewmen. Shackleton persevered for 14 months, in the end saving all against very long odds. How much more ought we marvel at Mandela, who persevered for more than 18 years, saving his entire nation!

Mandela shares the credit for this triumphant accomplishment, for he too was a learner, like all good teachers. He cites especially the influence of Mahatma Gandhi and Martin Luther King, Jr., whose own hearts and minds helped forge the insight and power that Mandela brought to Robben Island. They were crucial parts of his lineage.

Later, as my tour group drove in the bush along what could only satirically be called a road, our guide suddenly stopped the Land Rover and looked intently down at the road-side. "There"—he pointed—"rhino," indicating a fresh track. It was there—we could see it. But he had been driving at 25 kph. How could he possibly have spotted it? He stopped again, staring into the distance. Then he looked with binoculars. "Yes," he affirmed, pointing into a valley in the far distance. "There they are."

We saw nothing. But when we used the binoculars, we could just make out some small grey dots near a watering hole. A Londoner in the group exclaimed: "How did he do that? I couldn't spot a double-decker bus at that distance!"

How is *this* possible? The guide had highly refined detectors—powers of perception that seemed unavailable to the rest of us. When we inquired about that, he explained that he uses all his senses, all the time—that the air smells different if an antelope has recently crossed the road, that a few blades of grass at an odd angle are signs one can read, that a speck of grey in an otherwise green landscape or a rustling sound from the bush are clues. Hearing this did not enable us to do what he does, yet we were changed by that hearing, by that reminder of how underdeveloped some of our own potentials are.

We were not suddenly able to see rhinos, or even busses, a mile off, but we started attending in new ways, seeing more. Instead of just looking around, we were self-conscious about how well we were seeing. We smelled the air, scanned the grasses, scrutinized the distant views, listened intensely. Our heightened sensibilities enriched us, made us more fully present in and connected with our natural environment.

This is like Mandela's bequest to us. In seeing the humanity of his oppressors, he displayed rare moral discernment. He was more fully present in, and more fully connected with, his moral environment than what we typically think is possible. He thus enlarges our own moral sensitivity, our sense of the possibilities of moral discernment.

When we lose patience in the face of small disappointments, or lose grace in the face of real affronts, or lose hope in the face of seriously discouraging challenges, we might do well to recall this model of courage and moral leadership. It reminds us of what we could be at our best.

We have lost Mandela, but we need never lose the lessons his life has taught us. He will remain part of our own legacy, if we understand that enhanced noticing and empathetic reconciliation, rather than the demonization of others, are the best means to a peaceful future.

Theo—who fled Vienna before Kristallnacht and escaped the Holocaust—sought a peaceful future in every way he could. He was a strong defender of Israel—where his acting career had begun—but of a just and honest Israel that opposed being victimized by discrimination and equally opposed being the perpetrator of discrimination against others. He supported collaborative music projects that were developed jointly by Palestinian and Israeli artists in his lifetime, and his legacy now includes a foundation that continues to support such collaborations (www.theodorebikel.net). Like Doc Edgerton (of Chapter 12), he was all of a piece—not sometimes a singer or actor and other times a social activist. Whatever he did, he did with all his interconnected resources. He could focus on the one person before him and also see the structures and patterns in which that person's life and history were imbedded.

Despite his great success, Theo said he felt like a refugee ever since fleeing from Vienna. On the seventy-fifth anniversary of Kristallnacht, he was back in Vienna addressing the full Austrian Parliament, including their military leaders. He told them he had long wondered why he had been spared the annihilation that befell so many millions of others, and he conjectured that perhaps it was so that he could return on that occasion to affirm that the Nazi murderers were all gone, but that he was still there to bring a message of survival and peace. He played his guitar and sang for them and closed by blessing them with a prayer in Hebrew. The prolonged standing ovation could not undo history but was a gratifying step toward reconciliation and healing.

The present war in Ukraine would have seemed eerily familiar to Theo. In his autobiography (1994), he wrote:

My grandfather still lived in Czernowitz, the provincial capital of Bukovina, the area in Eastern Europe where both my father and mother were born. Bukovina, part of Romania when I visited there (now part of Ukraine), had been the easternmost province of the Austrian Empire prior to World War I; as the Russian troops advanced, my mother's family had fled to Vienna.

He would surely have grieved for the carnage and eagerly lent his talents to sustaining the spirits of the Ukrainian people. He would have identified with the millions of refugees fleeing as his ancestors fled. He would have sought, and found, ways to join the battle to protect and preserve the people, traditions, and culture of Ukraine—much as his brilliant play *In the Shoes of Sholom Aleichem* protects and preserves the Yiddish language of Theo's heritage.

Many creative people are exemplars of excellence within their domains, such as science, business, or the arts. These three giants—Edgerton, Mandela, and Bikel—spread their genius in different ways, in different places and times. But they were alike in the most deeply important way possible. They were exemplars of *excellence at humanity*: of understanding what being fully human is at its best and in seeing and wanting to nurture that potential in everyone.

CODA: THE LESSON OF AGNES MARTIN

Like the works of Rothko and Rembrandt, paintings by Agnes Martin require intense, sustained scrutiny. Although Rothko's and Rembrandt's works are compelling at first glance, that first glance can't even hint at the richness and depth that reward the patient, probing viewer. Some of Martin's works, at first glance, are barely visible. Her highly abstract, meticulously crafted grids and patterns come to life only slowly, as each viewer contemplates the emerging images. Understanding this, Martin denied that she even made works of art. Instead, she considered the work of art to be what happens when a viewer interacts with her painting. No two viewers will have the same interactive experiences, so each resulting work of art is unique to the viewer. Martin prompts the scrutiny; the rest depends on us.

That's a useful way to think of what I have tried to do in this book. Each reader will see different things with which to concur or disagree, at which to yawn or chuckle. A chapter that seems to one reader not to have earned its space may prompt another to discern something more clearly, to revise an old opinion, or to have a surprising flash of creativity. If any of that motivates a reader to talk with someone else about a story I've told, an opinion I've expressed, or a recommendation I've made, I'd count that as a success. Part of what I want to convey is that a philosophical perspective is in many ways a conversational perspective—not a body of information to learn, but a process of dialogue that probes, challenges, disturbs, clarifies, and inspires. Telling true stories is one way to do that; I've told these stories here in the hope that some of them have done so for you.

OUTTAKES

The pioneering quiz show, *You Bet Your Life*, was hosted by Groucho Marx and ran on television from 1950 to 1961 after starting as a radio program. It was conducted before a live audience and recorded on 16-millimeter film, then edited to prepare the film for broadcast. The program director, Bob Dwan, and I became friends long after the program ended. Because he knew many of the great comedians and understood how they worked, I invited him to Syracuse University to give a series of lectures and conduct a master class on the craft of comedy. He still had the outtakes, and we screened many of them in a session titled "Groucho Uncensored." We explored the changing standards determining what could and could not be broadcast; what those standards should be was controversial. What was not controversial is that some fine material had been languishing in the outtakes. Remembering that, I've included here some passages I wrote while working on this book, but decided did not have a proper place in the text.

In Chapter 18, I mentioned different characteristics of decisions. A choice can be important without being difficult: seeing the house engulfed in flames, we immediately call the fire department rather than going for the garden hose. A choice can be difficult without being important: a patron in a restaurant annoyingly dithers at length about which of two favored items to choose. Whenever we face a decision, there's no avoiding it. Even doing nothing is a decision, although typically a bad one. The house burns down; no dinner arrives. Confronted by a difficult choice, people sometimes identify what factors matter to them (cost, comfort, safety, service to others, bonds of loyalty, etc.) list the pros and cons of each option, decide how much weight to give each factor, and then pick the choice with the best score. But if we are disappointed to see the winning choice, we commonly rearrange the weighting of factors so the choice we feel better about wins after all, and our analysis has just been a rationalization that gives a deceptive veneer of rigor to our decision.

In Chapter 21, I mentioned some experiences with job searches. When I was nominated for the presidency of a small, high quality liberal arts college, I knew the job would go to the interim president, who was their provost. Having me (and others) in the pool was just a pretense so they could claim to have had a national search with a diverse array of excellent candidates, all of whom were then surpassed, on the merits, by the one finally chosen. (This sham is common in academic searches.) My candidacy reached the interview stage, and I agreed to go for the sake of an enjoyable visit and to learn from the experience. I don't regret doing that, but I have long since regretted my failure to seize a unique opportunity. Their search committee did something clever that I had not seen before: they divided into two distinct teams and conducted the interview twice. I was pleased to have given them ideas they seemed to value, such as how they could make better use of their emeritus faculty. Only later—and too late—did I realize what I had missed. I wish I had, in the second interview, presented a persona completely unlike that of the first interview, with diametrically opposed positions on various important matters. It would have been a treat to imagine the later meeting of the whole committee, trying to reconcile the two radically different perceptions of one candidate. (It might have been something like the conflicting views of one patient at Beth Israel Hospital, as perceived by the surgeons or the internists.) I'd have wondered how long it had taken them to figure out the prank—like the writing professor finding "cantaloupe" in every one of his summer high school students' papers.

A helicopter rushed a shattered elderly man to the shock-trauma unit at Johns Hopkins University Hospital. With skill and dedication, over several weeks, they saved his life and oversaw his recovery to the point that he could be discharged. One physician asked what the plans were for his care after discharge, only to be told, "That's not our issue. Maybe he has a social worker." Horrified, that doc replied, "An 82 year old guy falls out a window and nearly dies, and we don't even ask how it can be that he fell out a window? We patch him up and say that's not our concern? What are we sending him home to? We should care about who he is, not just what was broken!"

Michael Scriven, a philosopher with vast intellectual reach, has had faculty appointments in many fields and at least nine universities in his long, geographically and intellectually nomadic career. Even in his 90s, he was a distinguished professor at Claremont University. From 1966 to 1978 he taught at Berkeley and then from 1978 to 1982 at the University of San Francisco. Coming from an immensely wealthy Australian business family, he had deep pockets, and lived in a magnificent apartment on Russian Hill in San Francisco with a stunning view of the Bay. When I visited him there, he eagerly showed me his new high fidelity sound system, which enabled him to rotate a directional rooftop FM antenna toward the transmission tower of station he wanted to hear and displayed the incoming signal on an oscilloscope. He redirected the antenna as I watched, and I saw on the oscilloscope that the signal became sharper. But I could not hear what was a tiny difference; my auditory discrimination was not that sensitive. When I said I couldn't hear a difference, Michael said he couldn't either, but it pleased him to know that the signal was optimized. He was like that; wanted each thing to be the best it could be.

The story I think I remember is this: Michael taught at Indiana University from 1960–1968. There, the student newspaper published something so threatening to the administration that they shut the paper down. He then rented space off campus at his own expense and supported the re-establishment of the paper as independent from university support or control. I've tried recently to find him, to check the veracity of that memory—but to no avail. Nonetheless, I think of that story as a noble defense of vigorous investigative journalism under threat.

In Chapter 13 I described my unsuccessful attempt to title a book *Doctors of Virtue*, which I wanted to do because in each of its two senses the phrase applied to the content of the book.

I've liked ambiguous titles, from Tobias Wolf's triply ambiguous *This Boy's Life* in 1989 to the new Historic Grounds Coffee Shop in Beaufort, NC. In titling this book *Illuminating Philosophy*, I'm finally getting my way, using a title with two meanings—each of which describes my intent and, I hope, the content of the book.

Also in Chapter 18, I described the ironic assignment to write an email with no *e*. In 1957, James Thurber gave us *The Wonderful O*, a fable about despotic pirates who invaded the island of Ooroo, seeking treasure, and banned the use of the letter *o* there. But they were ultimately overthrown by the will of the people, who affirmed that hope, valor, love, and freedom cannot be banned or defeated. This month (March 2023) the people in Tbilisi, Georgia, filled the streets and forced the withdrawal of an anti-democratic Russian-inspired government bill that would have ended independent investigative journalism. And the people in Israel filled the streets, closed the airports, shut the universities, and forced at least a temporary delay in Netanyahu's anti-democratic attempt to eliminate judicial independence.

Dear Mr. Nadeau:

As long as there is one upright man, as long as there is one compassionate woman, the contagion may spread and the scene is not desolate. Hope is the thing that is left to us, in a bad time. I shall get up Sunday morning and wind the clock, as a contribution to order and steadfastness . . .

Hang on to your hat. Hang on to your hope. And wind the clock, for tomorrow is another day.

—Letter from E.B. White to a Mr. Nadeau, March 30, 1973

ACKNOWLEDGMENTS

Every person who appears in these stories, named or not, contributed significantly to this work; I am grateful to them all. I appreciate the support and encouragement of friends, family, and colleagues at and beyond Syracuse University—a vast array. My many mentors, and those I have mentored, have been sources of invaluable substance and inspiration. A research leave from Syracuse University, with support for research expenses, was crucial for this project. I am also grateful to the Guggenheim Foundation, which rejected my request for support. The application process for a Guggenheim Fellowship is arduous and demanding. Of the approximately 3,000 applicants with whom I was competing, only about 6 percent were successful. But I was successful too, in that their demanding process is precisely what produced the conceptualization of this project and the plan of work that led to its completion.

I regret the omission of any names that should be here but are not. Those to whom I know I am indebted are: Teresa Adorjan, Peggy Battin, Debbie Berg, Rock Brynner, Jonathan Dee, Debbie Douglas, Charles Fried, Martin Gellert, Arne Glimcher, Judith Gorovitz, Ruth Grene, Alexia Garaventa, Charlotte Grimes, Shelly Gruskin, Alanis Hamblin, Roberta Hennigan, Elizabeth Humes, John Huss, Danny Kahneman, David Kaiser, Kathleen Kaminski, Neal Katyal, Tammy Kiesa, Brian Konkol, Bernard Lyall, Ruth Macklin, Susan McGuire, Cathryn Newton, Donald Provence, Carol Quinn, Kara Richardson, Carol Roberts, Heidi Robertson, Peter Robertson, George Saunders, Jane Schwartz, David Seaman, Henry Shue, Jim Sidel, Jennifer Spitzer, Jeremy Townsend, Diane Wiener, and David Wilk.

And heartfelt appreciation to Art Caplan for his imaginative and generous Foreword!

ENDNOTES

Chapter 4

1. Z. Bankowski and J. Bryant, eds., *Health Policy, Ethics and Human Values* (Council for International Organizations of Medical Sciences), Geneva, 1985, pp. 105–6, 303. (This exchange appears as published in the conference proceedings, including a few small errors in transcription.)

2. http://law.justia.com/cases/california/calapp3d/163/186.html (The Bartling case, also in 1984, established the competent patient's clear legal right to refuse unwanted treatment.)

3. This sort of anti-intellectual administrative wrong-headedness comes and goes. It gives way to more enlightened leadership, yet sometimes returns. A commitment to vanquishing it is always essential.

4. James Wood, "Is That All There Is? Secularism and Its Discontents," the *New Yorker*, August 15 & 22, 2011, p. 89.

5. Family historian Joseph Lurie, at http://www.jewishgen.org/databases/USA/gorovitz.htm

INDEX